Diary of a Hippocrate

Medical School Years

Twana L. Sparks, M.D.

Jane —

There's no one

like you.

T Sparks MD

VANTAGE PRESS
New York

The identifying features of persons involved in this book have been altered to protect their privacy.

The road to becoming a physician is fraught with difficulty and ambiguity. It can be the best of times and the worst of times. Dr. Sparks and I both found it an honorable and fulfilling path.

—Sylvia M. Ramos, M.D., FACS,
Breast surgeon, private practice,
Albuquerque, New Mexico

To
Ken and Juanita Sparks, for
teaching me to love learning and laughter
and
Rebecca Smith, for challenging me with
blank pages
and
Judy K. Williams, for helping me with
my life

Contents

Diary of a Hippocrate

CHAPTER 1

Dramatic Times

The mother threw her clawing hands into the air, screamed agonizingly, and fell to the floor in an absolute faint. The father held his face in his hands and sobbed, "Jenkins, my little poor little Jenky." Their handsome happy four-year-old was dead. Less than an hour before, he wasn't.

I was a third-year resident physician on trauma call, when my pager went off for about the twentieth time that afternoon. "Trauma room, stat" it beckoned, with the same emotional effect as sandpaper on teeth. Already running to the unknown, I slapped the beeper-silencing button with the thought, *Go to heaven,* in the traditional sentiment of my chief resident (last-year physician-in-training). He referred to the pager, not the patient.

Arriving at the emergency department, I saw the familiar nurses, technicians, and ambulance personnel hovering over a tiny form. Mechanically, I started through the routine: A-airway, B-breathing, C-circulation, D-deformity, E-exposure. Within seven minutes it was clear little Jenkins had dilated pupils (possible brain death), a severely fractured neck (possible paralysis), and blood in the abdomen (possible serious internal injuries). Within five minutes, we were in the operating room with my hand guiding a knife into the child's belly.

The attending (a fully trained and licensed specialist), Dr. Stache gloved to assist. "What's the story?" he asked as we placed retractors, suctioned blood, inspected organs. "Some driver didn't slow as he took an exit from the Interstate. He drove over one car and landed on top of the car this little guy was in. Seat belt didn't help him this time," I replied.

The liver was torn in half along the vena cava, the body's largest vein. Jenky's heart stopped about then, due to shock (low blood pressure) from blood loss or spinal cord division or brain injury. We spent another twenty minutes trying to start the heart, having pressure packed the liver and substituted a plastic tube for the vena cava. Someone muttered a trauma team maxim, "Sometimes dead means dead."

En route to the waiting room, I tried to imagine an acceptable way to break such news to the family. In a minuscule conference room with two low couches and subdued lighting, I could only come up with, "I'm sorry. We did all that we could."

When the mother regained consciousness, she was still screaming. I'd never lost or even had a child. I could not imagine the pain of such a loss. I offered to let the parents spend time with what remained of their son. As I led them toward a blanketed bundle in a corner of the recovery room, I contemplated how I had come to be in this horrifying, yet wonderfully privileged position. This is the story told in my journal, a review of four years in an ordinary life.

CHAPTER 2

The Beginning

Year One, August 2

Today I arrived in the place where I hope to fulfill a lifetime dream. I'm just four minutes' walk from the Emerald City, where the wizards of the body will surely teach me the secrets of life.

There must be a point in every life when a person decides what to become or else becomes something through indecision or default. If all kids grew up to be what they thought they wanted to be, there would be mostly firemen and ballerinas living in America. At age ten, I latched onto a heroic, romanticized occupational hope for a career in medicine. I was discouraged by several friends and considered nursing as an alternative, thinking I could not afford medical school. Yes, I would be a veritable Florence Nightingale! (More accurately, I think she should have been called Florence What-a-Nightingale, being rumored to have given syphilis to 50 percent of the soldiers under her care during the Crimean War.)

A love interest in college convinced me to abandon the nurse idea. We would become medical laboratory technicians together and try for medical school. The relationship didn't last, but the idea became a deep obsession.

I marched out, newly degreed, idealistic, applications in hand, at age twenty, only to receive a raft of rejection letters. I mourned for seven years, singing the med school reject blues. I'd been enhancing my life in the meantime, studying psychology, starting a rape crisis center, learning the banjo, working at a laboratory job that I'd hoped I would never have.

I tried again. The admission committee must have surmised me to be more mature, well-rounded, experienced, or something. I am fantastically excited to be here. It's better than the day God created Houston to punish man for his sins.

August 5

Why am I doing this? It will require total energy for five to eight or more years; then I'll have to be accessible to the public for the rest of my life. I want to know all I can. It will take a lifetime to ponder the complexity of the human body. How could I ever get bored?

I wandered through the medical school library today, perusing the stacks. I feel like a horse chomping at the bit; I'm so hyper to get started. Even the titles are exciting: *Pediatric Trauma, Medical Biochemistry, Pain, Holistic Health.* This is my opportunity to apply my hands and mind to real suffering with some tangible results. I have the chance of discovering something totally unknown, which could change the course of how the earth lives. I guess everyone has that chance; this just feels like the right niche for me.

Here's the second law of thermodynamics: All energy travels downhill (entropy). Healing, which the body does of its own volition, is a statement against that law. Isn't that great? I want to be part of it. This self-propelled process can repair some pretty incredible burns, amputations, crushes, etc., although not perfectly. It can maintain a sackful of chemicals and water upright and functioning for over a hundred years! The organization of the body seems to get more specialized and less repairable as it travels upward. For some macabre reason, I've been thinking of how much of the body can be removed and still leave a functional person.

Actually, all we need are our upper halves. Leave the head, arms, chest, liver, one kidney, and a few yards of intestine, and the hemi-person could still be independent, except for needing artificial means of mobility. I don't want to be that person, but I do wonder why I can replace miles of toenails and not one brain cell.

August 6

Spent the day thinking of all the people who made my being here possible. My hometown Latin American Club helped with my tuition, and I'm not even Hispanic. Friends and family shipped me off with well-wishing, cash, clothes, furniture. The physicians I had worked for during the last few years were just rude. When asked for letters of recommendation, one said that if I'd write it, he'd exert the energy to sign it. Another, my best possible reference source, said he'd write that I had come to work sober, on time, and done a great job in the lab, was conscientious and honest and good natured, but that "girls" didn't belong in medicine. I didn't ask him to submit the letter but did query him on when he thought I would qualify for womanhood, being twenty-seven years old at the time.

August 8

I hope my ultimate practice will reflect some of the idealism with which I am approaching my new work. American doctors have accomplished an incredible amount through discovery and technology. I am proud to be associated with that aspect. My exposure to them in general, however, has left me with a stereotypic picture of greed and arrogance. I know they, soon to be we, have special knowledge

5

and training and gave up many young years to get it. In return, I hope to receive a comfortable, safe home, food, clothing, two weeks vacation a year, and, if I earn it, community respect.

August 9

I couldn't help myself. Went to the library and got the book on holistic medicine. There is a bush, particularly abundant in east Texas, commonly called sienna tea. The brew of this plant is a powerful laxative. It can be grown and baled in such abundance that a fair commercial price would surely be less than an ordinary tea bag. It is used as a purgative before bowel X rays and sells for about $5 for four ounces. I don't get it. Why can't I give my patient a leaf, let him brew it, and save him $4.95? Perhaps I can learn about this too. Why is a tank of oxygen a certain price and, when the same tank is labelled "medical," the price doubles?

One of the reasons that occurs to me is the need to cover technological expenses through overcharging on medicines. Perhaps there are issues of quality control. Perhaps patients are more compliant if they have to pay more and something looks more high-tech. Only four more days till I start to get some answers, maybe.

August 10

Today, I learned that life is not a drug-dependent state. I never realized I was part of a society in which many problems are inappropriately solved by medicines. Can't sleep? Take a pill. Can't stay awake? Take a pill. Can't cope? Take a you-know-what. How come we didn't learn change your lifestyle, exercise, eat better, and quit drinking as solutions?

August 11

I am part of a fairly unique experiment in medical education. After the first month, I won't go to classes or take tests. I'll go to tutorials and do apprenticeships. The theory is that material learned in context will be retained. In other words, I'll remember eye anatomy and function better by being part of an eye examination and corneal transplant then by reading about them in six separate segments during the next two years. This approach is problem-based, student-centered, as opposed to subject-based, teacher-centered. With guidance, I am to solve medical problems by teaching myself, using the materials I choose. Isn't that a nice adult approach? I'm told I will learn as much and as fast as the traditional student, and it will stick. It will be enjoyable too, getting to ask the questions before I am given answers. Motto: What's learned with pleasure is learned full measure.

It seems very practical. An analogy would be a pilot who has read all the right books, made passing grades, understands the instruments, etc., then is placed in a cockpit and expected to fly well. I read *Problem Based Learning* by Howard Barrows today. I am so ready to get started on this!

August 12

Only one more day of being an unmedical student. I decided to learn about Hippocrates, to kill some time. I don't know if I will be asked to take his oath, but I'd like to know what it is.

Hippocrates' notes show extensive knowledge of ulcers, tetanus, fractures, childbirth, and much more. He lived about 500 B.C.

The Oath (with minor annotations)
I swear by Apollo[1] the physician, and Aesculapius and Health

and All-heal[2] and all the gods and goddesses that, according to my ability and judgement, I will keep this oath and this stipulation—to reckon him who taught me this art equally dear to me as my parents, to share my sustenance with him, and relieve his necessities if required; to look upon his offspring in the same footing as my own brothers, and to teach them this art, if they shall wish to learn it, without fee or stipulation; and that by precept, lecture, and every other mode of instruction, I will impart a knowledge of the art to my own sons, and those of my teachers, and to disciples bound by a stipulation and oath according to law of medicine, but to none[3] others. I will follow that system of regimen which, according to my ability and judgement, I consider for the benefit of my patients, and abstain from whatever is deleterious and mischievous. I will give no deadly medicine to anyone if asked, nor suggest any such counsel; and in like manner I will not give to a woman a pessary to produce abortion.[4] With purity and with holiness, I will practice my art. I will not cut persons laboring under the stone,[5] but will leave this to be done by men who are practitioners of this work. Into whatever houses I enter,[6] I will abstain from every act of mischief and corruption; and further, from the seduction of females or males, of freemen and slaves. Whatever, in connection with my professional practice or not, in connection with it, I see or hear, in the life of men, which ought not to be spoken of abroad, I will not divulge,[7] as reckoning that all such should be kept secret. While I continue to keep this oath inviolated, may it be granted to me to enjoy life and the practice of the art, respected by all men, in all times! But should I trespass and violate this oath, may the reverse be my lot!

If I were to take this oath, I would swear by gods with whom I am not familiar. I would promise to house old doctors, or at least support the Old Physician's Home. I very likely would not place a patient on morphine and water to meet the end more peacefully.

I do not know that I would ever perform an abortion. I have given much thought to this complex issue. I find it an unacceptable method of birth control. From a Judeo-Christian perspective, it seems a fetus was not the equivalent of a man, at least in the Old Testament. I deduce this from the comparison of Exodus 21:12 and 21:22. In the New Testament, however, dignitaries such as Jesus and John the Baptist seemed destined from conception to fulfill prophecies.

From a secular perspective, a Carl Sagan thought is worth contemplating: Because of the vast number of brain synapses,

> . . . the number of different [mental] states [possible] is two multiplied by itself ten trillion times. This is . . . far greater than the number of . . . electrons and protons in the entire universe. These enormous numbers may explain something of the unpredictability of human behavior. There must be mental configurations that have never been entered by any human in the history of mankind. From this perspective, each human being is truly rare and the sanctity of individual human lives is a plausible ethical consequence (*The Dragons of Eden*, reprinted by permission).

Notes

1. Apollo was the god of healing in Greek mythology.
2. Aesculapius was Apollo's son, one of whose accessories was, and still is, the rod or staff with the entwined snake on top. Another staff and snake symbolized safety or health in the Old Testament wilderness. It was held up by Moses, reportedly healing all who looked at it. Health and All-heal were Aesculapius's daughters, also known as Hygeia and Panacea.
3. Medicine as an esoteric study was, and possibly still is, being clung to as a realm for the select few. Hippocrates does offer to share it with the more serious and committed.
4. He tries to convey the sanctity of life concept. A pessary is a vaginal suppository. Many methods of abortion were known then, including severe bleeding, leaping from heights, dilation of the cervix, and use

9

of herbal stavisacre and mezeron pessaries, which were apparently successful.

5. One version reads, "I will not cut for stone, even for patients in whom the disease is manifest." It is unclear what this means. Is it kidney, gall, salivary, or bladder stone, or does he mean amputating parts to free a person?

6. Housecalls?

7. Confidentiality.

CHAPTER 3

Let the Insanity Begin

August 13

Orientation followed by emergency-medicine class at long last! The dean welcomed us with, "Medical school isn't as hard as it used to be. In past years, we opened with, 'Look at the two people on either side of you. Next year, one of them will be gone.' Now we try to help each person succeed." The competition will still be pretty cut-throat, I suspect, since top grades help secure a better residency (specialty training) program spot at the end of medical school. In the tutorial system, however, I will be graded by my peers on my ability to bring and present information, so there's no way to cheat or compete. What a concept!

The class is very diverse, with ages nineteen to thirty-six: Asians, Native Americans, Hispanics, and 36 percent women. Some are snot-nosed brats, some physical therapists, waitresses, even a few farmers. The adrenaline level in the auditorium today could run the world for a few days. I felt like every rotten thing that ever happened to me in my life was compensated for by this day. It was electrifying.

The reason we started on emergency medicine was explained by the dean. "Yesterday, you were lay persons. Today, your neighbors and acquaintances will think of you as doctors, so we want you to know what to do when the lady next door runs into your apartment with her child choking on a penny."

I bought and began reading my first textbook. The first paragraph is about air. If you ain't got air, it don't matter what else you got. Now I know the danger of a hole in the chest wall. The diaphragm pulls down, and instead of pulling air into the lungs, it pulls in air through the hole to surround and collapse the lungs. I learned about fifty other useful, interesting new things. This tidbit from a former veterinarian: If one lung gets collapsed by the method described above, a person can survive. Buffalo, on the other hand, have a single compartment containing both lungs, so a well-placed arrow to the chest wall can fell a mighty beast. I don't think I'll ever try to kill a buffalo, but now at least I know I need to hurry if I'm going to save one.

I am awestruck to realize I may act correctly in a crucial moment, allowing a dying person to walk away. Now my year would be set if I could find my fantasy book, *Biochemistry for the Feeble Minded*.

August 18

What a week! I walked across the lawn at my apartment complex to buy a newspaper. Some guy stepped through my unlocked door and welcomed me to the big city by stealing the billfold out of my purse. I even saw him walking away from the door. I haven't really got time to replace my driver's license, credit and Social Security cards, figure out which check number I was on, and I'm not too happy about the lost thirty dollars that could have fed me for a week. The first day we were told to plan on studying seventy hours a week, which I have tried to honor. I resent having to spend any spare time I have atoning for my acts of stupidity.

August 19

During lecture today, about twenty people with paper

bags on their heads came running, screaming through the lecture hall, throwing candy at us. Then a few marched through with a banner reading "Welcome Newcomers." The prime innovator of the problem-based learning project had all twenty of us in the experimental group over for dinner and orientation. The other fifty-five people in the "regular tract" are variously jealous and ridiculing. I am supremely happy with my present lot in life.

August 21

There has been a lot of posturing and false bravado displayed as many of my fellows try to show they are the cream of the cream of the crop. Several professors have addressed the issue while the two segments of our class are still together. One gave us some advice along these lines: You people have probably never failed at anything or you wouldn't be here. You were the football captains and first-chair trombonists. Start preparing now to fail with some patients. You will miss a diagnosis, make some terrible mistakes. Your only consolation will be that you did your best. Try to truly learn the material, not just memorize it.

Another ventured to guess that the majority of us had a hidden fear that we were not as good as the others around us, that we had somehow arrived in this prominent group by mistake. I certainly worried about it. I'm older, out of school longer, never heard of Phi Beta Kappa honor society, have no relatives who were doctors. Then a wonderful thing happened. The emergency-medicine block grades were anonymously posted, and mine was the highest. All the "kids" are speculating who is such tough competition.

August 24

What is the world's most dangerous drug? I'd say it's a

tossup between power and alcohol. The latter has more to do with my immediate focus. I've been making a list of interesting alcohol facts revealed to me in the last few days. Other names by which it is known are ethanol, booze, hooch, CH_3CH_2OH, the scourge of mankind, the two-carbon fragment.

Concerning snake bites: Fifty percent of all people invenomated are intentionally handling the animals and 50 percent of those are drunk and have impaired reaction and/or judgment.

Altercations: Many persons severely injured in fights are too chemically altered to defend themselves.

Freezing to death (hypothermia): This occurs generally when body temperature reaches 94 F (34.4 C). There have been recorded survivals at both 79 F and 51 F, however. The intoxicated person feels warm and often falls asleep outdoors in dangerously low temperatures.

Inhibitions: Part of our survival is based on our inhibitions against death (suicidal and accidental) and pain. Alcohol lowers these inhibitions.

Slow suicide: Sufficient years of alcohol intake will produce liver cirrhosis and brain damage and plasma buildup abdominally and agonizing death. Other gifts it imparts are pancreatitis, gastrointestinal hemorrhage, seizures, behavior disorders, central nervous system failures, broken lives, broken homes.

(Hope I haven't bored you with this page, but I needed to record that the problem is so pervasive and serious that it boggles the mind. I forgot to mention that 85 percent of auto accidents are booze related.)

Why is alcohol such a problem? I'm sure the answer is complex. My answer is that our general populace sees the "two-carbon fragment" as fun, food, and/or consolation, but not as an extremely dangerous drug.

That statement reminds me of a quote, author unknown

to me, which proposes, "Complex, difficult questions have simple, easy-to-understand, wrong answers."

CHAPTER 4

Walk a Mile in My Shoes

August 28

The final week before the class splits into traditional and problem-based tutorial tracts is over. It has been a fabulous time, with so many new people in my life with whom I have so much in common. The curriculum made a noble attempt to teach us how to communicate with outpatients. We had a short course in counseling and interviewing with lots of role plays.

Some highlights were guidelines on how to be nonjudgmental, nonthreatening, nonauthoritative, and understanding. Of course, being judgmental, threatening, and authoritative are some of the things I do best, so I was pretty much lost. I wasn't the only one. At least I had a concept of how to be understanding. Patients have begun to rebel against being treated as sick objects. Diagnosis requires a knowledge of the stressors acting on a body, or so says the holistic approach. For a person to share his/her work, familial and personal emotional problems with a doctor, s/he must trust. We tried to learn how to show total acceptance. It seemed to me the jocks (athletes) of the class tended to resort to pep talks, flavored with "get a life, grow up, quit whining" advice. It was fun, and I learned a lot about myself.

I was in a group of eight people who did role plays all week. A few had trouble recognizing feelings, as in wouldn't know one if it broke in and ate the EKG machine. The three who I thought were the least talented at it all turned out to be children of physicians. Whoa, what's that all about?

I was assigned to play the role of a forty-eight-year-old Mexican-American man who, after suffering testicular cancer, has just been told it has spread to the brain, without hope of a cure. This was a fascinating and terrible exercise, to try to mentally cross gender, culture and age barriers to imagine his reaction. The threat to his masculinity, the helplessness of leaving seven children behind, the pain and fear of dying so young were nearly overwhelming, even to me in my remote position.

Other people played a sixteen-year-old girl who has attempted suicide due to pregnancy, a seventy-year-old Navajo woman who can't keep food down, a ten-year-old boy whose whole life is running track, who has just sustained a debilitating injury in a wreck. We then went to area hospitals and interviewed willing patients.

In the remote past, medical students learned this way, by doing. Now, it has become the tradition for them not to see patients until the third and fourth (so-called clinical) years. Seeing them in the first month opened a huge world of thinking to me. Medicine has become more than challenging, more than trying to contribute something to society. It is testing one's mettle against all the problems, pain, and death common to humanity. When success occurs, internal rewards are incomparable.

I began training with a volunteer group called the sexual assault response team. We will aid doctors in collecting evidence from and offering counseling to rape victims. I have some experience with this, and it is easy to get burned out, focusing on the senselessness of it all. I keep picturing an image of one of the cases I "worked." The scene included a young woman in a white uniform, with her slacks and underwear beside her and a bullet hole in her temple. It doesn't need any explanation. Rape is not a sexual crime; it is a crime of violence. This society seems to thrive on violence in all forms. We use it for entertainment, problem solving, and gratification. We seem to adore and condone it. This absolutely must change; we must raise children who can relate to other people in healthy ways.

Since the 1950s several things have been available that are new to humanity, partially accounting for our lack of interactive health. The most important is the widespread popularity of the electronic babysitter known as television. The content of the programming is probably much less important than the fact that viewing substitutes for human interaction, which is how we learn about functioning well in society.

A second new powerful event lies in the availability to children of enormous amounts of information that is not filtered through older and presumably wiser, guiding, loving minds. The information is filtered by those in control of the media instead, whose main interest is promoting consumerism and entertainment, or reporting horrifying occurrences, which are adult worries.

I knew that The Three Stooges didn't really poke each other in the eyes. I don't think the generation surrounding me misunderstood what was real; I think many didn't have enough meaningful human contact to care whom they poked in the eye.

In my life B.M. (Before Medicine), I volunteered at a rape crisis center. I also did an extensive survey in a small community to determine the occurrence of rape there, including males and females. Canvassing those eighteen years and older by anonymous questionnaire, I found an astonishing 30 percent of the women reported having been raped. One out of every seven men said they had been raped by other men. I started a rape crisis center there, since the need for support seemed so enormous.

This has been a heavy week, a "touchy-feely" experience of gut-wrenching magnitude. I gave out some awards on the last day to try to lighten things up. The woman who portrayed the ten-year-old in the car wreck had wrapped a few of her limbs with toilet paper to heighten the effect. She got an Oscar for "Best Special Effects." One fellow received a certificate of creativity for having conducted his real-patient interview while seated on her portable bedside commode.

Interspersed with all the rest of the curriculum, there was a quick review course in statistics, or sadistics as I think of them. I'm not great at most forms of math. Although I battled my way through calculus to get here, I still can't get my checkbook balanced.

September 2

Five students, in a tutorial with a tutor (basic science professor or M.D.), get a case story, decide on who will address which "learning issues" by the next meeting. There's a loose organization in which we usually (1) identify the patient problems, (2) hypothesize what might be wrong, (3) rank order and test the hypotheses.

We decided early on that our first patient had heart or lung trouble. Someone was to bring back information on the anatomy of the heart. I've seen the plastic models, colored the thing in my anatomy coloring book, even held a dead one in my hands, but still was having trouble with understanding the dynamic motion involved. Our lecturer for the day (alias fellow student) made a controversial revelation, that the right external jugular vein imitates the behavior of the right atrium (first heart chamber). There was a fair-sized argument, which the tutor resolved by standing all five of us in a circle, assigned us to be parts of the heart, and moved us through the entire cardiac cycle. I was so honored to be the controversial jugular vein. Next week, I hope to present the lungs as a one-act play.

After that we went to lunch. I think we are enjoying ourselves more than the other fifty-five who are sitting in a cramped lecture hall, scribbling notes, dreading their first examination.

September 8
Someone found my wallet, sans the thirty dollars.

September 9
We went to the runaway shelter today for another patient interview. The people there are some of the most vulnerable in our population. Most have been rejected by parents, attacked by strangers, and abused by peers. Most of them need some medical attention; they live in a war zone.

Two new friends, Rave and Mary, and I played with the heart model for an hour. It would take a Ph.D. in engineering to get it back together. Rave dubbed it "Rubik's heart."

September 10
Something is happening to me. It's a fullness I can't describe. Maybe it's equivalent to a manic phase or a prolonged peak experience. Everything is wonderful, being exactly where I want to be, doing what I must have been meant to do. All the simple pleasures of life are suddenly so poignant (dear God, perfect oatmeal, once again!). I bet I'll get over it.

September 12
The euphoria continues. I feel as if I am living with the

people in my tutorial. Much of what we have learned so far has been about dealing with each other. It is already an emotional obstacle course. In the group, I've jumped from angry to omnipotent to foolish to competitive to bored to numb to ecstatic in one morning. This has great potential for personal growth, and it is practical in teaching us to communicate with peers and patients, family and mates. We actually say the words, "You're wrong," and "I don't know," without anyone being devastated. This learning program is pretty ambitious.

September 13

Medical school is not so much difficult as it is voluminous. Here's what I learned (taught) today: In the body, amino acids (small proteins) are the building blocks, and sometimes can be transformed into each other. Phenylalanine is such a block; most of it is converted by an enzyme into tyrosine. In phenylketonuric (PKU) babies, the enzyme is missing. Most American babies in the past twenty years have been tested for this problem. Since phenylalanine cannot be converted, it builds up and begins to poison the brain. If we keep eggs, meat, and dairy out of the diet while the brain is growing (about six years), retardation and death can be avoided.

About now, the first PKU babies have grown to reproductive age. Since the diet is relaxed after age six, these mothers have phenylalanine in their blood, which is harmless to them, but poisoning their offspring at the rate of 90 percent. The congenital retardation seen in the second generation is a doctor-caused disease. In one generation, there will be more PKU-related retardation than there would be if the original researchers had just left the problem alone.

Now there is a new problem being addressed: How can surviving "normal" PKUs reproduce without producing retarded children. Four proposals have been made. First, re-move the mother's egg, fertilize it in vitro (outside the body) and implant it in a healthy woman. Second, keep all PKU females on the diet until conception years are over. Third, start the PKU females on the diet and prevent conception until phenylalanine levels are normal. Fourth, sterilize them all?

The disturbing conclusion is that doctors and medical researchers can make the quality of the genetic pool of humanity, hence the future health of generations, poorer with each passing year. We are gradually eliminating the survival of the fittest. Persons with hemophilia, cystic fibrosis, Hunt-ington's chorea, sickle cell anemia, and many other diseases are surviving to contribute to the human DNA definition. Duplication of the weakest is now possible for the first time in known history.

I'm not implying that persons with hereditary illness have any less right to survival. They obviously have the right to have children, but they are born with a greater responsibility in their reproductive decision making.

I wager no one will quiz me on these philosophical gems, but they will expect me to know tyrosine converts to melanin, a major pigment in skin and hair. since phenylalanine cannot convert to tyrosine, all PKU babies will have light-colored hair. Now I have to go memorize the chemical structure of all the amino acids. I think there are twenty-one.

September 19

I have been officially introduced to my cadaver. Students in the traditional tract began on day one, instructed to start dissecting at the shoulder, proceeding in a systematic removal of deceased layers. The special students, such as my lucky self, go to the cadaver lab to answer specific questions relevant to the cases we are pursuing.

There seems to be a badge of honor given primarily to medical students; we are allowed to cut dead bodies. The bodies of paupers are no longer used for our "scientific purposes" and each person lying there is self-donated. In the lab are about thirty metal tables, each with an occupied body bag. The embalming and other preparation (head-shaving) cost about $2000. I don't know why.

There's no special immunity to being nervous or somewhat repelled by death by virtue of having started working on a cadaver. I know the obese woman in her fifties upon whom I practice my awkward craft was someone's daughter, possibly wife, sister, or mother. Her remains deserve the same respect as a body undergoing any surgical procedure. There is an eerie atmosphere, however, and a lot of probably inappropriate things are being said. One member of the team is having such an emotionally hard time, due to lifelong superstitions, that another member of the team is considering arriving early in the lab, hiding in a body bag adjacent to our table, and then planning a struggle to free himself from the bag after we arrive. The plan was canceled when we suggested to the prankster that the fearful one might suffer a cardiac standstill, and we didn't have a defibrillator handy. Someone named our cadaver Abra (Abra Cadaver).

Obese people are hard to examine, in life and in death. Alive, I can't hear their lungs, feel their livers, locate their breast lumps. In death, I keep destroying the very things I am seeking, since most of the veins, arteries, and nerves are encased. To make it more difficult, surgical adhesions are slowing us down. Sometimes, when we arrive, the object of our search has been heisted by some surgeon years before.

23

September 20

Could not study any more. Spent an entire evening playing music and singing with some old friends who were in town. If one is accepted into medical school for being well-rounded, there isn't much chance to express it there.

September 24

Finding less and less time to write. Before medicine (a common phrase, abbreviated B.M. by some of us), I was a letter writer. Now, my time is too short, so I will be xeroxing my journal to send to family and friends.

Trouble in paradise! Our tutorial is really having growing pains. We meet three times a week for three hours. The members and tutors will change every two months. At the end of each session, we evaluate each other concerning information given, and ability to communicate. Sometimes it is great fun, but this week three members have been clashing over facts and personalities. Much of our time has been spent learning to deal with people, as opposed to learning to deal with appendicitis.

Went to the pediatrics clinic to do another of my interviews. Took a syringe to offer as a toy, but it turned out my patient was only ten days old, and not much interested. Her mom really liked it; she was fifteen. Also, had my final interview with a nursing home or "elderly care center" patient. Summing up her problems, I'd say grief and loss were at the top of the list. Her life is so different from mine, with loss of health, home, children, coherency. She's tried to make the best of her world. When I presented her to my group, the only term I could find to describe all her health complaints was "organ recital."

Received my bone box today. It's a dismantled skeleton for use as a learning tool. Sure is complex, with all its bumps and dips and landmarks. I guess "the hip bone connected to the thigh bone" won't get me by. He's been dubbed my Marginal Man.

On my way to mid-tutorial evaluation tonight. It's a dinner, followed by two hours of assessment. It will probably get even more intense than the short ones in tutorial, and I have to evaluate myself. It is a form of exam. There are written exams in the problem-based curriculum, but they amount to practice board exams, and I take them at my leisure to identify my weaknesses.

The organization of medical training in America starts off with two years of classroom, followed by written boards. If one jumps through that hoop successfully, two years of hospital patient contact are followed by another set of boards. If that labyrinth is successfully maneuvered, one is called Medical Doctor, taa daa. Then, in most states, at least one year of internship is required for a person to open a general practice office. General practice is my present plan, since I am a little old for lots of years of specialty training. I'll have to see what fits me.

Another type of test we have in our peculiar system is case problem. Each student is sent into a room with a patient (real or actor) and has an hour to complete a history and physical. This will be observed through a one-way mirror. Then the student (namely me) will have forty-eight hours to "solve" the case and write it up. Then I meet with an evaluator, and explain all my reasoning or lack thereof. This test is given after each two-month tutorial. I think it's a very realistic way to test physician skills.

CHAPTER 5

Sights and Sounds

October 1

Evaluation was pretty painless, at least for me. The tutorial group wound up reprimanding a couple of people. One for sulking and one for passive aggression. The first stopped sulking and became a true pleasure to work with, and the latter got more defensive, childish, and cruel. Mixed in with all of this, we were still able to learn about the function of the liver. Only a few more days of this group, then we all get new groups!

Started a new sort of meeting/learning session. We are learning to do physical exams on each other. It was easy to do heart, lung, extremities, nervous system, and abdominal. The lessons today were male genitalia and female breast. At the beginning of the week, we were informed of the anticipated class, and asked if we would give permission to be examined by our peers, or if we would prefer to have the school hire models. Nearly every one volunteered to be a patient, so those of us who were reluctant felt pretty prudish and agreed as well. Only one male abstained, and a tutor volunteered to be his substitute.

It was difficult to be clinical with our newfound friends and enemies, but all survived. It was so successful that I got to discover a supernumerary (extra) nipple, varicocele (varicose vein of the scrotum), and see a student, who also happens to be a nursing mother, demonstrate the fact that she could write her name on the wall in human milk. She epitomized how comfortable people were with the whole idea by the end of the session.

I'm getting so good at this that, if I cut my nails, I could set up a hernia diagnosis booth at the mall.

Walking to school, I heard a soft intermittent hissing sound over my head several times. The neighborhood dogs were barking wildly. I couldn't see a thing until it passed in front of me, my very first hot-air balloon. It was blue, a world globe, with beautifully colored continents. Next a sky writer started doing his smoky thing. I'd never seen that before either. What would it be? Something romantic or something profound, I was hoping. But no, just McDonald's.

Getting home, I encountered a bearded, bruised, WASP-ish-looking guy wearing cut-offs and Indian war paint, shaking a leather strip with bells on it. In the other hand, he shook a brown beer bottle with a rock inside, and did a rain dance for about two hours at the west end of the apartment complex.

Sometimes I believe the whole world is solely engineered for my amusement.

October 7

My remaining grandfather died this week. I flew out for the funeral, and had to rush back to another reality so I could perform my first end-unit exam. It was hard to concentrate on the test, and I didn't find much comfort in the funeral, so canned and ritualized. Seems to me churches and hospital chapels and mortuaries need areas set aside for screaming.

My test was videotaped and critiqued. I figured out the most likely diagnoses and treated appropriately. The only negative comment was, "Don't tell the patient, 'Hope for the best.' If you want to relieve anxiety, try, 'I'll be here to help you through whatever this is.' "

Someone rigged an old ammunition box into a bomb at my complex and left it by the dumpster. A curious passerby opened the lid and is in intensive care full of metal pieces. While hearing this news in one ear, I could hear, in the other ear, organ pieces from a twelve-hour Bach-a-thon at a building across the street. Seems such diverse occasions of horror and sweetness could not coexist in the circuitry of the same brain without producing at least a schizoid personality, if not worse.

October 26

The latest adventure is a trip each week to a prison farm to do sick-call for the inmates. I also will be working in jail and greater security prisons. The electives are quite varied, so I chose one I thought was most foreign, so I could learn the most.

The nurse at the honor farm clinic spent a great deal of time explaining that the men would fake illness, get angry, manipulate the staff, and make passes at the female students. The preceptor/tutor later said, "In six years of doing this work, the only time we've had problems was when the guards made passes at the female students."

I was quite nervous, though. I am still new at doing such intimate things to strangers, and I had a vague fear of being taken hostage by nightfall. I thought it went great and said so at my self-evaluation later. I had to confess one interaction that I could have managed differently. I was doing a physical on a man in his forties. After he dropped his pants for the genital portion, he said, quite sincerely, "I'm sorry about the hard-on. We don't see many women around here and none of them touch us at all." Hoping to offer some professional response, I formulated several possibilities in my racing mind. Such things as "Don't worry about it" or "Forget it" seemed okay. Unfortunately, what issued forth from my mouth, to my dismay, was, "Oh, I hadn't even noticed," which I suspect was not the least bit comforting to him.

The tutor advised us all to read something relevant, so we might understand our patients' lives more clearly. I picked up a book written by a now free inmate, *The Hate Factory,* by W. G. Stone.

The most disturbing part of the system is the behavior code among inmates. For example, if one sees a rape, or gets raped, and reports it, the most abhorred transition takes place. The witness is then wearing an imaginary "snitch jacket." Other inmates will no longer interact with the snitch, and he must be isolated for his protection. Someone in his family may be punished outside the prison, or his life and limb may be in danger upon his release. Almost any behavior is acceptable, because no one is going to complain.

Others who must be placed in protective cells are the child molesters and the weak (physically or mentally). Prisoners believe in capital punishment. During riots, they generally torture and destroy those living in protective cells.

October 31

Went to a Halloween costume party in the middle of the day, thrown by a couple of tutorial groups. My costume took an hour. It was a bed sheet shaped into a cone, with green balloons pinned all over. It was a fair representation of a bunch of seedless grapes. Rave came as a box of Tylenol. We went to the cadaver lab to harass the regular students, since they have no control over their schedules whatsoever, and couldn't come.

My new tutor, Will, offered to trade me a passing grade for my costume. I declined the offer, but gave him the suit anyway, since my party was over. My black tights didn't fit, so he ran out to buy some Big Mama panty hose. I think this anecdote and the photos may be of use later.

CHAPTER 6

This Stuff Is Hard

November 3

Learning much of the material is similar to acquiring a foreign language. I heard we learn an average of ten new words per day. The pages of my histology (cell structure) and biochemistry books are stuck together with blood, sweat, and tears. It is difficult to see the relevance of some of it. The wonder of it all continues when I am privileged to uncover, for example, how bone can heal, solid as rock, yet be alive!

December 20

The books are calling so loudly that I have had to be unfaithful to my journal for a while. I am trying to run thirty minutes a day, so I don't lose my health completely. Several of us decided to start, but we don't run together. We talk about our endeavor in derogatory terms, because none of us are very athletic. We are not very fast either, so someone named us the "Half-fast Running Club." It's a pun.

Here's a little consoling anecdote about a Doctor Fisher, the man who discovered the structure of the glucose molecule. He had to carry his notes to the chalkboard when lecturing, because he could not recall the structure of the thing and neither can I.

One of the inmates told me, "I hate the Southwest part of the country, because of how inhumanely they have treated me here. Once I heard a story of a sailor who began to hate the ocean, and didn't want to have anything to do with it again. He never wanted to be reminded of it. He put an oar over his shoulder and began to walk inland until someone pointed to the oar and said, 'What's that?'

"This is what I'm going to do when I get out of prison: tie a huge taco on top of my car and drive until I hear somebody shout, 'Hey, what is that?' That's where I'll settle."

January 12

Learning this month about venereal disease. The old gold standard, syphilis, is known as the great masquerader. It could be the pain in the joint, the dementia, the rash, the deafness, or any other presenting symptom. An ad in the local college newspaper reads, "Male herpes victim wishes to establish relationship with similarly infected female." Since it isn't curable, this approach seems incredibly socially responsible. Something that seems totally new is Acquired Immune Deficiency Syndrome (AIDS). It is an unknown force that knocks all the fight out of the immune system.

The primary theory behind AIDS at this point is very odd. It proposes that the immune system is "overwhelmed" by too many infections. This sprang from the fact that most of the affected are homosexual men who have had many other infections, such as syphilis, tuberculosis, amebiasis, hepatitis (A, B, non-A, non-B), gonorrhea, and giardia (an intestinal parasite). The human immune system is so infinitely versatile that it is difficult to imagine it just fizzling out. Another theory involves a communicable virus, which would make it potentially the next Black Plague.

In times past, persons with fatal, communicable diseases, such as TB or leprosy, voluntarily secluded themselves to protect those around them. This type of personal responsibility has probably been replaced by a demand for individual rights. One of my hospitalized gay interviewees told me he would be willing to go to such a place, trusting that it would be one of the most party-filled and best decorated-places on Earth. Another told me in prison that AIDS is known as PB (which stands for parole board), as it is a very certain indication that a prisoner will be leaving prison earlier than anticipated.

One of the gonorrheas brought back from Vietnam is not sensitive to any antibiotic. It's all very depressing and very preventable.

January 18

I got to do my first small surgery today. It was only opening a little infected cyst. My preceptor showed me how to inject, incise, drain, and bandage. For some reason, it was a terrific thrill. As a medical technologist, I drew blood, assisted with autopsies, cared for people's ailments indirectly. Now, I have the honor and responsibility of caring for them directly, and I actually helped someone on the road to recovery today. It has the potential to be fairly messy (birthin' babies comes to mind). The reward for digging around elbow deep in foul body fluids is that people seem to get better.

January 21

2:00 A.M.. I can't sleep. Took a break from school, for some entertainment, and went to see the movie *Gandhi*. Maybe I should have chosen something a little less intense. Never having been a student of world history, I am completely overwhelmed by the story of his life and concepts. I want to know how to reconcile the idea of the nonviolent man with a society that revolves around professional football, game hunting, and that mega-game, war.

I want to know what I can do, armed with the new knowledge of the fact that there can be enormous good, even in the power of one. I can go bury myself in a poor community, and be totally self-sacrificing, or be ambitious and cash oriented, and bestow it on needy causes. There are lots of combinations in between. I don't have the vision yet to know where I belong on the continuum.

A lot of people recognize me on the street because I have seen them as patients. I feel bad not recognizing them. I may be their only doctor, but each is only one of about a hundred patients I have seen.

In all the weight of learning, one of my cohorts, Ron, is a bright spot, always with a distorted, disturbed outlook on any question. The current tutorial was discussing how to test the first cranial nerve (smell). It is inconvenient to carry coffee grounds, or cinnamon and such, in order to be thorough. Ron's suggestion was to complete the rectal exam with one's gloved finger, have the patient close the eyes, then see if they can identify the odor on the finger. He is truly disgusting, and makes such long serious, acquisition of knowledge more tolerable.

CHAPTER 7

Out to a Wider World

February 22

My heater pilot light went crazy and burned up the appliance. The smoke alarm let me know, but I didn't have a fire extinguisher. The fire department only took five minutes, but a maintenance man had cut off the gas by then. I don't want to die by fire.

March 21

Apprenticeship started today, in the small town of my choice. I started shadowing Dr. Morton. It is fascinating what he does all day. Saw a proctoscopy and sessile polyp near the valve of Houston. I'd hate to be that anatomist, Houston, and be remembered for near eternity for a mucosal fold in the rectum. Now I have to go home and find out what it all means. I plan to learn one drug per day, and review it with Dr. Morton, and again and again as we use it. It's an almost painless way to learn pharmacology.

First drug du jour was thyroid. The thyroid pill turns out to be just that, pig thyroid. It's reassuring to know that in case of nuclear holocaust, a guy on thyroid medication can still obtain the necessary supplements, provided he can find a farm or weiner factory.

March 25

I did a paracentesis today. Yesterday, I didn't know what one was. Here are the steps: Do a sterile prep. Tap on the abdomen, to see where the fluid level is. The bowel is full of air and floats to the top. Insert a needle and draw off a liter of fluid caused by cirrhosis of the liver. Stand back and watch the patient breathe better. It's cookbook style. It's dangerous. It's temporary.

April 1

What a great week in pediatrics! Newborns are different from other humans, in many more ways than their total dependence. They have different reflexes. Their bones and skin and heartbeat are all distinctive. They have a big hole in their heads. They throw up all the time and survive. Their abdominal muscles are so thin that one can feel the tiny muscle band at the stomach outlet. They like being held by the jaw, with their breastbone resting on a larger person's forearm.

April 3

Even my obsession with medicine wanes occasionally. Took a night off to play guitar and sing corny old folk songs with two really nice guys. Cleaned the house. What a relief to do anything that wasn't medicine.

April 4

Setting: Examination room.

Characters: Pediatrician, parents, eleven-year-old girl, social worker, first-year medical student observer.

Plot: Child is physically precocious, looks sixteen, been having menstrual periods since age nine, is now pregnant.

Doctor gives the parents the bad news, waxes eloquent about pain, anger, support, etc., discusses counseling with the social worker.

Disturbing flaw: Nobody once addressed the child.

April 7

One conclusion I can draw after two weeks of doctoring kids is that it's pretty scary owning a body. It is really hard to get personal information out of them. I think the adolescents are afraid they will be reprimanded or they will seem stupid for worrying about something trivial.

One teenager had a growth on his arm for two years. It was discovered in a routine sports physical. He had developed another on the forehead, which he was growing his hair long to hide. We sat down to tell him and his family it was a cancer, probably incurable. I asked him why he hadn't said anything about it. He really couldn't respond except to say he was scared.

April 8

I thought medicine would be pretty routine here. There is no such thing. Every diagnosis is a puzzle. This week alone, we are "working up" a child for tropical fungus infection, maybe even a lung fluke (flat worm). Her family just came back from a vacation in the South Pacific. I saw a man whose only symptoms were sore fingers and toes and a variable fever. He has an infection of a heart valve, which is throwing off little bacteria bundles, which are lodging in the hands and feet. It could be fatal or cause a stroke if it wasn't identified early. The next day, met an eight-year-old who had suffered a stroke from the same illness.

A woman came in with complaints of itching for over a year. She has tried changing her laundry soap, diet, job, husband, and everything else she could think of, with no relief. Dr. Morton thinks of a rare liver disease—that sends bile salts to be stored in the skin—runs a few liver tests, and Bingo. The amount there is to learn is overwhelming.

April 12

Flew to a rural clinic with one of the family practitioners. The physician's assistant there has a television camera to transmit videos of patients and X rays back to the main office 125 miles away for advice.

April 14

Saw a child come into the world today. Although it is everyday, everywhere, it was much like my experience with death, rare and awesome. We are so protected from witnessing these wonders in our society. The pain and the joy, the energy and the exhaustion, the father's love as he sat at the head of the table with eyes glued to the mirror over us, the blood, the tears, the anticipation, and finally there she was, Lakie!

April 16

Had supper with old friends. I brought my ophthal-moscope (eye-looker-inner thingie) as a conversation piece. Both Becky and Trevor found the optic nerve, which is really difficult. Ptolemy, the cat, had an astounding rainbow for a retina (lining of the back of the eye).

April 22

Got to stitch up a foot in surgery. This is some of the most exciting, interesting, and enjoyable work I've ever done. It doesn't feel like work, actually—more like Disneyland. There are several of my peers who find it totally boring, even vile. It is wonderful to do something manual and be able to stand back when it's completed to see the finished product. It is less satisfying (to me, at least) to give a prescription, encourage a lifestyle change, do a little education, and sit back and wonder if any of it will make a difference in the life of the patient.

May 1

"Assisted" in a cholecystectomy (gall bladder removal), which means I held retracting instruments so the surgeon could see. It took a hard, constant pull for forty-five minutes. I think I'm more sore than the patient. My reward for this was closing the skin. The trick is to get the needle into dermis (second layer of skin), pull closed, lay down a snug knot (approximate, don't strangulate), and the incision should meet, dermis to dermis, in a nice neat line. Mine looked similar to the Grand Canyon, but steri-strip tapes made up for my lack of skill.

May 4

Trying to take care of a schizophrenic gentleman who keeps running through the hospital naked, trying to get back to the woods, to live "simply." Wish I could let him.

May 14

We must be having a special on psychotherapy this week. Everybody has the crazies. Master manipulating hypochondriacs, and manic-depressives, and eating-disordered people with no self-esteem and a few unprovoked hostile patients to boot. One forty-year-old had a "positive review of systems." He had every single symptom I asked.

"Headaches?"

"Yes, very bad, right here," indicating entire head.

"Ringing in the ears."

"Yes."

"Shortness of breath?"

"Yes."

"Diarrhea?"

"Yes."

"Constipation?"

"Yes."

I tried to present him to Dr. Morton, but could not come up with a physical diagnosis that encompassed all his complaints. Morton said, "I want you to go back in there and ask him two more questions. If you get affirmative answers, the diagnosis will be easier."

What a genius this doctor is, I thought. "Tell me the questions, please. This patient is very confusing."

"First," he said, "do your teeth itch? Next, do your stools glow in the dark?"

May 18

Obese people are so hard to examine and treat. I learned thoracentesis (chest cavity fluid removal) on a very large woman today. The concept is to numb an area to one side of the mid-back, find a pair of ribs lying over fluid, and slip a needle in to drain it all and let the lung fill up its proper space. First, the poor woman's back was so thick that I couldn't percuss (hear by tapping) where the fluid level was. Then, having estimated the level by X ray, I couldn't feel any ribs through all that insulation.

My drug of the day is a blood thinner, coumadin. It's been the most widely used for thirty years and the cows discovered it. They were eating some spoiled sweet clover up in Wisconsin, and every little injury made them bleed profusely, because they couldn't clot their blood. The substance was isolated, mixed with ground glass, and used for rat killer. Now there's a pleasant way to leave the world, don't ya know? It was considered too dangerous for humans, but someone tried to commit suicide with it in 1951, and didn't die. Thanks to his failed attempt, millions of people have survived deadly disorders of overclotting.

May 24

Hey, one of my patients has the plague. Some flea off some rodent probably jumped on her while she was outside playing. Then a bubo (lump) swelled up in her groin and she got a fever that won't respond to penicillin. As long as it's bubonic plague (with just buboes) she isn't contagious. If it becomes pneumonia (pneumonic plague), she can infect us all with a cough. That sums up the Black Death of the 1300s.

The plague is rare in America, but rather common in Asia and South America. People all over the world are dying of this and many other treatable diseases, like tuberculosis and leprosy. I wish for a world without borders, political, financial, or medical, but don't know how to create it. There's a popular T-shirt here, which includes the zia symbol from the New Mexico flag and a pertinent quote, "Land of the flea, home of the plague."

June 17

The home office sent out someone to check on my progress. They call him a "circuit rider," and he came to check my records of what I say I have learned here. I'm making good progress.

The pediatrician is on vacation, so I went shopping for a specialist to teach me something. The ophthalmologist was willing, so I milked him for information all week. Watched the repair of a torn tear duct. It was really delicate. Went home and learned the anatomy. Not surprisingly, even tears are complex, with three layers, oil, mucus and water. Missing any component of them can mean a dry eye and blindness.

June 19

Assisted with a stillborn's autopsy. The cord had gotten wrapped around the neck so tightly that the brain did not receive its fair share and quit sending impulses to the heart, which quit beating.

Then, I went to the hospital to watch another birth. The parents were so happy when Lynn Kody slid into this life, that everyone in the delivery room cried. This profession is such an emotional roller coaster.

June 25

I am house-sitting for someone this week. They have a lot of animals and pet birds, and a VCR. I'm renting about ten movies and have a marathon film festival with some friends who are having a birthday. They are Marla and Karla, what you might call "wombmates," or twins.

June 27

The party was a blast. Much to my chagrin, I have discovered the house and my body are infested with fleas. I can't really spray without taking out all the birds. It's too much trouble, so I'll just stay at my place, and go out for mail and animal feeding. I called a fellow medical student, Greg, to get some input about my newly acquired parasites. He was quite informative, told me someone in California had tried a flea collar. Dogs have no skin pores, so the insecticide is harmless to them, but on humans it soaks in. The Californian had lost his life in search of better hygiene. Greg suggested I shave half my body, and when the fleas jump to the bald half, I could kill them with an icepick. What a great guy!

June 28

Helped put an arm back together. An elderly man fell through a plate glass window, severing many muscles, exposing bones, but miraculously not injuring any nerves that allow for hand use. His family placed a tourniquet, probably saved his life. We put another on in surgery, and released it every so often to see where the worst bleeders were. There is, for limbs, a "golden eight" hours, during which they can do fairly well without circulation. My time here is almost done, and it's back to tutorial time.

June 29

Very excited to be going home. I'll pick up one of my nephews, the four-year-old, for a few days of fun. I like to grab one of them once in a while, just to be around a healthy kid. Speaking of unhealthy, saw a baby this week whom the doctors don't know whether to label male or female. Genital development is so complex. I learned that all embryos start out physically (not chromosomally) female. When testosterone starts being produced, the male embryos begin to differ. Some male embryos do not respond to the testosterone, and go on to become females externally, but males internally. They are not usually identified until puberty, when they fail to menstruate. This, and all sorts of other arrangements occur. The present child has what are termed ambiguous genitalia. So, till the chromosome studies are back (XX=girl, XY=boy) and the surgical possibilities for matching physique with chromosomes are evaluated, the parents are in an uncomfortable

43

limbo. They have given the child a unisex name,* and don't know what to answer when asked the gender.

*Pat, Chris, Terry, Kim, Leslie

CHAPTER 8

A Little Vacation

Year 2

July 23

I love my dad, though he doesn't talk much. He took me fishing last week and bought a ticket to the beautiful Cayman Islands. He doesn't have cash to spare, but he wanted to congratulate me in a big way. I hope my many siblings don't mind. I have been trying to study seventy hours per week. It is highly motivating to realize every fact absorbed may be useful in saving a life, or relieving some suffering. Fear of failure is also highly motivating, as is desire for approval. I'm sure they all play roles in my ability to focus, but I need a big time break. Wonder where the Cayman Islands are. Maybe I should ask someone so I'll know whether to pack a swimsuit or parka. I'm too tired to bother, so I'll take both and get on the airplane.

August 8

I went to the tropics. I slept and slept. I didn't read a single word except a menu. Broke open one of the multitudinous coconuts, ate it in the nude in the afternoon rain on my private hotel balcony. Thought maybe I was dead and in Heaven.

I ate conch and turtle at the "Grand Old House." Got

flashed by a construction worker and was too disconcerted to use my sister's line, "Looks like a penis, only smaller." There actually is so little crime that no one locks cars or houses. I was offered lifts every time I walked, and gave several hitchhikers transport on the day I rented a car. The people are friendly and cheerful. There seems to be no unemployment, taxes, poisonous snakes, mosquitoes, racial prejudice since it was settled by blacks and whites who intermarried. My landlady at the hotel had me over for dinner. Fried plantain was a new experience. She told me there is a blood disease common there, due to the limited population. So it isn't exactly paradise. It is pretty difficult to get citizenship there, despite the inbreeding problems.

I snorkeled off Eden Rock, a seventy-foot mound of corals, so rare and breathtaking it is impossible to describe. I'm ready to immigrate.

Met a guy with cerebral palsy (I guess) who had spastic movements of everything in, on, or around his body. His buddies called him Wobbly, which he thinks is a great compliment. As Wobbly got more blitzed on beer, he tried all the harder to play pool and sing with the jukebox. I never saw anything funnier or more human in my life.

September 7

What a hammering schedule, no time to wax eloquent. We were all asked to assess our personal development during our rural experiences last spring. My creation follows.

The Integration of Life and Medicine

Since this appears to be a highly personal and philosophical assignment, I'll address it that way. To answer the question as to how to integrate life and medicine seems to require a recognition of why I went into medicine at all. The two main purposes were to do good for my fellow humans, and to be all that I can be. There's a conflict between those two ideas, in that the first demands selflessness (I will go to school for what seems like an eternity, I will stay up all night delivering babies, etc.) and the second demands self-interest (I want to run an hour a day, I want to make music every day, etc.).

My rural preceptors taught me a great deal about how to accomplish both to a reasonable degree of satisfaction. Before, I had trouble justifying meeting my own needs, thinking of them as selfish. The concept of "self-interest" as opposed to "selfishness" was never clear to me before. I understand that a physician must maintain his or her mental and physical and social health in order to function well professionally. Unfortunately, each person is given only a limited amount of energy.

If a person sacrifices sleep too often, s/he'll do poorly during the day. In medicine, the easiest way to protect against exhaustion is to work in a partnership, allowing time for refreshment and a break from having always to be accessible, affable, and able.

Albert Schweitzer moved to the jungle of Lambarene. His life was medicine, I suppose, but he still took his organ and played concerts.

Another hurdle in the integration of life and medicine is the tempering of idealism (what I thought the practice of medicine should be) and realism (what it is). There is cause for great disillusionment for young physicians. As a medical technologist, I envisioned I was saving lives and alleviating suffering. That may sometimes be so, but in American medicine, whatever one's position, most of the time is spent trying to save people from their own self-destruction rather than some invading microorganism. The drunk who wrecked his car killing three innocents, the coronary patient who ate and smoked his way to heart failure, the hypochondriac with liver pains are all suffering from a common ailment: disease of low self-esteem. My conversations with my preceptors practicing

47

rural medicine have been invaluable in helping me view self-destruction as a disease to be dealt with as any other. Now I can combine medicine and REAL life, as opposed to my previous untenable goal of treating the ideal life with ideal medicine.

The joy and wonder and intensity of what I have been privileged to see and do as a doctor-in-training have allowed me to feel more fully alive and more purpose in that life than anything I have ever done. I have to keep in mind that being a doctor is not all that I am, nor all that I do.

CHAPTER 9

Still Excited

September 16

Something new to do. We must watch three autopsies, and submit a research paper about the cause of death to the chairman of the pathology department. The only way to make an "A" is to teach him something in the course of the paper. One of our best students, Caryn, reacted to that statement with, "I wonder if he knows how to tap dance?"

I'll be doing my jail elective again and, in the Spring, escorting high-school students through the emergency room, to see the results of substance abuse. Many patients are willing to be interviewed and become examples for the teens. I may do some follow-up research to see if such an approach to education about drugs and alcohol—that phrase is redundant—has any effect.

Still bashing away at tutorial-style learning. It is logical, exciting, and pleasant, for the most part. The instant friendships available have proved to be a first-rate support network. I was surprised today when someone hired a female stripper for our tutor's birthday. She was quite good, even tasteful, if one stretches the imagination. What was really great was the sophisticated tutor joining the spirit of it all, dancing with the pseudo-showgirl while she did her thing. He was pretty artful, flinging his beeper to the left, his watch to the right, one shoe to the ceiling. Thankfully, the cake showed up while he was working on his shirt.

These ridiculous scenarios make the days more tolerable.

September 17

I forgot to record what our class did to welcome the incoming novitiates. On their first day of class, I expected them to be pretty antsy. I didn't know what the traditional students had planned, but I showed up at their invitation to be part of the welcoming committee. We were all issued body bags and little bags of candy and stationed at the back door of the lecture hall. I climbed into the bag, pushed my legs through the plastic so I could walk, and waited for the signal. As one of our cohorts entered the front door of the hall, pushing a gurney holding an occupied body bag, we silently filed in the back. The freshmen were preoccupied with the scene before them and didn't notice us.

In a few seconds, whoever was playing dead up front began hoisting a carrot-sized object perpendicularly at groin level. As the newcomers began to realize their "corpse" was having an erection, it also turned on a tape player, blasting out the music to a popular song called "Science." After the initial confusion, there were hoots of approval for the trick, and we fired our treats at them as we ran helter-skelter through the room.

September 20

Reported on autopsy case number one, a man in his thirties who died suddenly. It's such an odd feeling to know he was eating breakfast with his family, and an hour later I was wandering through his heart chambers trying to learn what caused such an untimely death. Perhaps the answer will lie in the toxicology studies (blood and urine screens for poisons and drugs).

Five prominent medical educators came to take a look at our experimental-learning tract. We got to be the focus for a week and meet some academicians whose textbooks we've been using. One very congenially told us we are all going to be scientific illiterates. Fortunately, during one of my demonstrations of how the rural preceptors juggle their time, I got to hit the doubter in the head with a beanbag.

September 30

Had an end-of-tutorial case evaluation. My evaluator reprimanded me for avoiding the main issue (drinking) and using terms the patient couldn't understand (hypertension instead of high blood pressure). Live and learn.

October 15

My new tutorial is gung-ho on bringing in outside speakers. I think we're getting tired of doing all of our own research. We had a cardiologist and a nutritionist last week. This week, it was the Gay Speakers Bureau. There are two bath houses here, which I'd never heard of. We asked if they were not worried about this disease called AIDS. It is still unknown whether it is caused by a completely overrun immune system (seems unlikely) or a virus.

Almost to a man, they said they worried most about hepatitis, and that AIDS would not become a very large problem. I conclude that denial ain't just a river in Africa.

One made a point in contradistinction to an opinion recently expressed by a prominent but ignorant clergyman, who stated Acquired Immune Deficiency is God's punishment for homosexuality. Since there has never been a clear case of one woman transmitting any venereal disease to another woman, lesbians must be God's chosen people, the speaker noted.

The concept of sexuality is a highly complex and emotional one. There's a waiter/waitress here whose gender is absolutely indiscernible. S/he stirs up a lot of curiosity, but I wonder why. It seems we should relate to each other as humans, not gendered beings. I don't know why someone's gender should matter to me unless I'd like to have an intimate relationship with him/her/it.

I have categorizations for sexuality that I have never heard or read elsewhere. There are three types and four expressions of those types.

Choose one from column A, one from column B, and one from column C in describing yourself.

	A	B	C
	External Identity	Internal Identity	Fantasy Identity
Heterosexual			
Homosexual			
Bisexual			
Asexual			

A. External identity: How do you behave physically?

B. Internal identity: To which gender are you attracted? Which gender are you in your thoughts?

C. Fantasy identity: Which gender are you in your dreams and fantasies, and which gender is/are your partner(s)?

Now try to explain why you are any of those. Use bar graphs and percentages as needed.

October 30

Three hours of ecstasy at a Peter, Paul, and Mary concert. I wonder if there are any cultures with no music. What is it about melody that is a necessity of life?

Five guitar pickers came over to a housewarming since I moved to a new place, in a worse part of town. Can't afford the nice complex anymore, where my wallet was stolen and the bomb blew up. It was either move to the student ghetto, or get a Gucci flak jacket.

November 5

Studying on weekends for my national boards. There are many irrelevant facts that must be placed in long-term memory. I'm hoping I won't be like the constipated termite; he couldn't pass his boards, don't ya know?

November 6

Wrote my paper on the second required autopsy. A four-year-old girl with epilepsy had had a seizure while bathing in about four inches of water. She drowned. The way the pathologist knew she had a seizure was the bite mark on her tongue. I learned to caution parents of seizure-prone children about this possibility. I got an "A" for teaching Dr. Bigshot that it is virtually impossible to drown in the Dead Sea due to the extreme buoyancy. Also it is possible to dunk one's head while swimming in the Dead Sea, and cause laryngospasm (prolonged closure of the vocal cords) and experience a "dry-land drowning." It is possible to swallow so much of the Dead Sea water that the magnesium essentially paralyzes the body, and it may be mistaken for dead. All of this information is in the medical literature, but I would have to go to the Dead Sea for myself before I believe it.

While at the medical investigator's autopsy suite, I observed part of another case, a nineteen-year-old woman, hands tied behind her back, stabbed over and over, and add 140 more overs. I know from the history of the holocaust, European royalty, and the American West that man is capable of the most horrifying inhumanity to man, but to see examples of it firsthand is always a fresh horror. There are few people working at the autopsy office who oppose capital punishment.

January 12

Taking practice national boards again. If I do poorly, I'll consider forking over $800 for a Kaplan review course. I know I'm learning enough medicine to take good care of people, but I must cram tiny details into my head to score high. This will increase my chances of landing a prime specialty residency, they tell me. I'm not much interested in that, but it's two and a half years away, and I may find a different niche than I anticipate.

Seeing lots of patients in heroin withdrawal at the jail. Alcohol withdrawal can be fatal, due to seizures, but heroin withdrawal is not fatal. The classic symptoms are runny nose, runny bowel, muscle cramps and aches. It's like a powerful flu. We give them methadone, even though the misery only lasts three or four days. I don't understand the rationale. They are a captive audience and have an opportunity to break an addiction.

January 25

I passed the fake boards! That takes a lot of pressure off for the next few months. The real thing is in June, and determines if I proceed to third year.

April 4

Can't sleep, may as well write. We are writing our own cases now, choosing areas of identified weakness. My case is about poisoning. There were two toxins involved, lead and barbiturates. Lewis Carroll's phrase "mad as a hatter" came from the fact that people who made felt hats had to use a form of mercury that often affected their brains.

Downers (barbiturates) are fascinating, in that they stop breathing. If someone breathes air into the poisoned person, until the barbs wear off, full recovery is expected. If no air is provided, the heart is damaged by the oxygen lack. Remarkably, the brain is protected from cell death by this heavy sedation. It seems impossible, since the brain is the most delicate tissue of all.

Hypothermia (cold body core temperature) can have the same effect on the brain, so one must be careful in declaring cold and/or drugged persons as dead. Cold protects all the organs.

April 9

Took some high schoolers through the emergency room. They were overachiever types, who claim to have no contact with the drug crowd, so I don't know if it will have much impact. Several junkies warned them to just say no. One patient was a nondrinking bartender who was struck by flying glass.

I tried to temporarily anesthetize the neighbors' dogs. They bark incessantly and I couldn't stand it any more. I've spoken to the owners; now they haven't been home for days. I wasn't very brutal, didn't try a bottle of aspirin in hamburger, or something more sure. I actually wanted to throw a chloroform-soaked rag over each of their Doberman noses and hope for a few hours' sleep. Unfortunately, this technique of anesthesia requires a minimum of patient cooperation. I hung over the fence with my toilet brush and dripping rag, trying to use my throat as bait, but they both snubbed me.

My brother suggested barbiturates in Alpo, to produce a painless end. First, they'd probably get agitated, foam at the mouth, and fall over as good as dead. I decided I couldn't live with myself, but he pointed out that when they started foaming, the owners would decide they had rabies and do them in anyway.

May 16

The minutiae memorization continues in anticipation of boards. My favorite sample question so far has been:
The flagellum of a bacteria rotates

A. Clockwise
B. Counterclockwise
C. Both
D. Neither, it whips

How about E? Who cares and what does it matter? Or F? Clockwise but only in the Northern Hemisphere.

June 1

The real boards were more ridiculous than the preceding example. The flagellum question, or a variation of it, was there. Now, a few weeks wait, and I'll know.

June 15

I passed, what a relief. My scores were dead-center average, which is okay by me when the competition is stiff and I'm an educational experiment.

CHAPTER 10

Halfway Done

Year 3

July 5

Wow, what a horrendous schedule of obstetrics. Rounds start at 6:30 A.M. I have to see all my patients before rounds, so I can present them to the hierarchy of residents and attendings. Hematocrits (blood levels), blood pressure, and temperature are always good to know, especially if they are abnormal. Then clinic, or delivery room, or surgery until 5:00 P.M., then rounds again until 6 or 7, often staying all night on call till noon the next day.

I think there were more expectant women in the clinic today than I have seen in my whole life. Of the twelve I interviewed, ten had no means of support and eight didn't want to be pregnant. It's a sad commentary on our clientele, and on our society if this is a microcosm.

Discovered a different type of stethoscope that's on a metal arch that fits from the back to the front of one's head, and sticks out from the forehead. Somehow it is easier to hear fetal heart tones with this kind. I heard twins today; they have their heads between each other's ankles. Felt like a unicorn all day, searching for those little thumpers.

July 17

My notes are getting more fragmented. Here's a surprising tidbit of information: A lot of what we do is based on what we think is true instead of what we know is true, because we'll never know.

I'm trying to learn about Cesarian section. When a pregnant woman has active herpes, there is a 50 percent chance the child will catch it, coming through the birth canal, and 50 percent of those babies may die of the infection. Therefore, we deliver them by Cesarian. When the bag of waters breaks, the virus starts swimming upstream. If it has more than four hours to swim, we assume the baby is infected, and do not subject the mother to Cesarian or C-section.

July 30

Delivering my first baby was exactly what I expected: enthralling, amazing, and as frightening as anything imaginable. Those poor creatures mashed and contorted for hours, then someone grabs their little skulls, or some other body part, and pulls them into the cold, cruel world. It is all in the timing; can't do anything too soon or too late.

I brought three into the world this week. I only deliver girls, apparently. The reactions of the mothers have been varied. The first turned to her husband and said, "I'm so sorry." That one made me sick. I'll bet mother and daughter both have a great life ahead.

The second mother looked at me and asked what race "it" was. That one made me laugh. The last turned to her husband and said, "Thank you, oh, thank you. We made a little girl. Oh, thank you, God, thank you, Tony. Isn't that the most wonderful thing in the world?" That one almost restored my faith in humanity.

Yes, it really happens. A forty-year-old overweight woman,

a "grand multip" (greater than six children), with irregular periods, came to the clinic with a "bellyache" and delivered baby number ten on the clinic exam table. The astonished medical student sat down to do his examination and was clever enough to identify a crowning head. Made me glad I had chosen door number one, since she was behind door number two. I might not have been as insightful and could have precipitated some disaster.

A twenty-year-old from Laos with lousy blood-cell levels was found to have two intestinal parasites and a liver fluke. We can't treat the parasites for fear of harming the little one. I was astonished to find she has no idea where her husband works or what he does for a living. My supervisor says that's not so unusual in lower socioeconomic groups. Makes me wonder what the couple talks about.

July 29

I have been thinking about becoming an obstetrician. Even if I go into general or family practice, I'll need to know about gynecology. The department asks all students to at least observe a "P.I." (pregnancy interruption), also called "T.A.B." (therapeutic abortion). There are steps involved that one would need to know if removing a fetus that had died, so it is an educational experience, in a manner of speaking.

My observation day was very draining. It was a suction approach, and my job was to search through a few ounces of debris, to make sure all the "parts of an eleven-week fetus" were out. The ribs, the tiny hands, the heart as small as the pupil of my eye, were all there. My heart was breaking for all the people who have gone through this, all who are sensitive enough to suffer over it, and more so for those who are not sensitive enough to suffer over it. I do believe there are people who should not be raising children, but I favor some other alternatives.

August 3

Assisted with surgery on an interesting benign (nonmalignant) tumor. In the abdomen, a cell, probably an egg, starts growing and makes a bunch of disorganized, but differentiated (specialized) tissue. It's a cyst that takes years to get to a noticeable size. On excision, the teratoma (monster growth) may have hair, a tooth, skin, etc. The one we removed had a tooth.

The surgery prompted some resident to tell a story from his medical school days. On trauma rounds, a woman involved in an auto accident had an abdominal film done. It was being reviewed by an entire team of doctors and students. One resident was quite proud to have noted a tooth in the lower abdomen and was waxing verbose about how it was most likely a teratoma. A medical student mumbled from the back row, "She must have a pretty aggressive dentist." The resident hadn't noticed that the tooth had been filled. The woman must have swallowed it when she struck her face on the dashboard.

Spending over a hundred hours a week in the hospital. What a joke to try to go home and study. The way I learned to teach myself in medical school really isn't a possibility with this schedule, yet. Maybe I'll figure out a way.

August 20

Sat with a woman through labor today, "helping" her push. It's one of the jobs of the medical student in the labor and delivery unit. Seems like such a waste of time, and I never got the feeling she really wanted any help pushing, or felt support from some stranger. I held out through my stint. She was rushed off to delivery about the time one of the patients I have been following in clinic came crashing through the door to have her triplets by C-section. I went to assist and never knew if my little pusher had a boy or girl or did okay.

The triplets were beautiful, and lasted long enough in the womb to have fairly mature lungs on arrival. Three identical girls. That's all I ever deliver, just girls. I'm done now with obstetrics and gynecology, and go on to pediatrics.

August 21

And who are my first patients? The triplets. They are still named A, B, and C. I'm also taking care of a little noodle with a cleft lip. It is so hard on the parents. I'm sure every parent carries in his or her mind the picture of and hope for a perfect child. When a newborn has a defect, there is an obvious grieving over that lost imagined child.

September 11

Pediatrics is proving to be mostly social problems. Kids get sick, or fail to get well around here, because adults don't take very good care of them. They eat cigarettes butts. They roll off the coffee table at age three months, and other silly things.

September 30

I have concluded that I won't be adequately prepared for general practice after medical school, and should go on for further training. It is all enjoyable, but I don't know if I have a special talent for a particular segment of medicine.

October 9

Internal medicine rotation has been raging for a week. I'm not as good at it as I want to be. I'm rushing through the "workups" on people who have always got more than one problem. Dr. Morton made it look so easy. I guess he knew many of his patients well and didn't have to reiterate their illnesses if they were unchanged. These poor patients see a different medical student every week, and each of us starts all over. I still have no clue as to how to advise, convince, cajole, or educate my patients into taking care of their health.

October 30

I'm getting faster and more focused with an "H&P" (history and physical). In fact, I'm an H&P factory. We third-year students spend much of the day running errands around the hospital, gathering results of tests, and getting equipment set up for procedures. This labor of love is called scut, and we are called scut puppies (a.k.a. scut dogs, scut monkeys, scut boys and girls) and we must "run scut" to have meaning in our present lives. We also calculate fluids in, fluids out, write progress notes, admit notes, discharge notes.

Another term of endearment/abuse employed by a particular resident is "newt," as in an immature salamander, signifying our worth, hierarchical position, and place on the food chain. Another label is "docklings," since we follow the real doctor around like so much poultry. Each afternoon, we hear on the overhead paging system, "Dr. Newt to the fourth floor," and all the little docklings come running, bringing their scut treasures. One student actually detests the newt label and is lodging formal complaints. Personally, I believe 90 percent of life is absurd. Only love and and death deserve serious consideration or reaction. The newt label falls in the

absurd category and should be treated as such. In psychobab-
ble (sic), it just doesn't push any of my buttons.

The jargon and abbreviations are so frequent that I
needed a translator for the first week. For example, the resident on call began my first day of rounds with, "I was hoping
for a no-hitter, but got slammed by a train wreck last night,"
which means, "I had hoped for no admissions, but received a
person with many serious problems requiring much attention."

December 5

I am rotating at a veterans hospital. Money seems to be
no object here. Many patients seem to use it as a hotel. It is
very frustrating work because it takes so long to get anything
done. An EKG and chest X ray can take all day. Then the
technicians can't find them to be reviewed. The nurses are
spread so thin that I don't know how they can survive. Someone told a joke on rounds: "How can you tell how long a
patient in this hospital has been dead? Count the number of
food trays in the room and divide by three."

Veterans have given so much to this country that it is an
insult for them to receive the kind of care available here. I also
consider it an insult to be asked to give this kind of care. Free
care is not synonymous with good care. I understand people
have been raging about this system for years, so I don't expect
I'll be able to make much difference, but I will look for a way.

December 23

The attending for this rotation has been unable to answer
the majority of questions posed to him, and the answers have
ultimately proven to be incorrect. He is not able to advise the
residents on any matters requiring judgment or experience.
The medical students were allowed to evaluate his perform-

ance, and vice versa. On my evaluation, he continually referred to me in the male gender, made erroneous statements
about my performance, and clearly hadn't a clue who I was or
how I had done. That's my grade for two months hard labor.
I, and all the other students, gave him failing marks, and asked
that he never be allowed near another patient or student. He
was promoted.

January 12

I'm on the downhill side of this all-consuming project
now, at least in my mind. In the next few months, I must decide
what kind of physician to be. I don't have enough information
to make that decision yet. I may never get to do a rotation in
dermatology; how do I know if I am perfectly cut out to be one
of those? I like almost everything.

Most third- and all fourth-year students are discussing
how to get the residency of your choice. Some say you must
be in the top tenth of the class to land a choice position.
Others say the top 10 percent are thought of as bookworm
intellectuals with poor patient skills, who don't make good
coworkers.

January 20

Oh, no! I love surgery! My stereotype of surgeons is
arrogant men with a lousy bedside manner, and there certainly are some of those. When I am in surgery, I have the
feeling I am *doing something* for the patient. It's not a pill and
a pat on the back and a prayer that the patient will comply
with at least some of my requests. Maybe the attraction has to
do with being in control of the situation. The patient is
unconscious (compliant), and more depends on me at that
moment than depends on them. The guy with the hernia
repair still has to have strong enough tissue and a heathy

enough nutritional state to heal, and can't go home and lift weights right away, but I have done something. It is usually immediately gratifying. Those near death from a ruptured appendix get up and go home in a few days. The blind see, the lame walk. It's so concrete. It's so bloody. It's hurting people to help them.

January 24

I am back at the Veterans Administration Hospital (VAH). This place is so disgusting. I'm not referring to the physical place, although it has what I call a fecal-nicotine veneer on the walls. Every inch of it smells the same. The more repulsive part is the way it is run. I went to help in the orthopedic clinic today. The hand clinic to be exact. It takes about three months to get an appointment in the hand clinic. About thirty people (veterans) waited those three months. Most drove fifty to three hundred miles, or flew or rode a bus, to get there. The hand attending didn't show up. Just me and a first-year general-surgery resident. I doubt if someone who actually knew something about hands could have done justice to thirty people in one afternoon. I know we two untrained people didn't. Rumor had it that the attending was helping with some orthopedic emergency. I'll never know. Surely someone with a little experience could have been sent in. I get the idea that these patients just don't matter.

I'm taking care of an inpatient who rolls himself out to the porch to smoke. He's on oxygen. Oxygen is flammable. He caught his oxygen tubing on fire, just under his nose. Now, besides his other problems, we are treating him for smoke inhalation and second-degree (partial skin thickness) burns of the upper lip. It happens to someone here about once a year. Maybe some of these patients don't matter to themselves, either. One day I expect the tubing will blaze on down to the

66

oxygen tank on someone, and we'll see him rocket over the entire building.

January 29

It's a little difficult fitting in on the surgery team, being the only woman. A lot of the decision making and information sharing is done in the locker room, apparently. In midafternoon, the gentlemen find thirty minutes to go "shoot some hoops." I never go, mostly because I'm never invited, am only 5'3", and never could hit the basket, and I refuse to lead cheers.

Today we did a colostomy takedown. It's the reversal of the operation that creates an opening on the abdomen, over which the person must wear a plastic bag to catch bowel movements. I asked the attending, a large, stern-faced, world-famous surgeon why the operation was being performed. He replied, "The joys of colostomy are overrated."

The "boys" on the team thought I was in big trouble for not knowing why we were doing the surgery. Then they thought my goose was cooked when the attending asked me a question, which I was unlikely going to be able to answer. Careers are made and destroyed at such moments in the life of a medical student. Impress the right person, and one may have an advocate in times of need. Fail at such a moment, and a feeding frenzy, with the student as lunch, may ensue.

The question went something like this: "Tell me, almost Dr. Sparks, how many people die as a result of their colostomy takedown operation? What percent have a fatal complication?"

The answer to such questions is either 15, 50, or 85 percent. I thought I'd better be honest. "I don't know, sir."

"Well, then," he continued, "if you had a colostomy, would you want it taken down?" Now the question had been

67

personalized, and I certainly would like to know my odds of survival, but I still didn't know, so I opted to be funny. One never knows if this is a safe course, but it was already clear that I was ignorant on the point.

"Would I want my colostomy taken down? I guess that would depend on if I had to mention it on my computer-dating form." The attending boomed with laughter. I don't think people play with him much. "Sparks," he said, "I think you have the makings of a surgeon."

It was a good day. My definition of a good day: Nobody yelled at me and nobody died.

January 30

Assisted with a skin graft. We took a skin cancer off the chest, patched it with thin skin from the thigh. There is a meshing machine that cuts hundreds of tiny slits in the skin graft so it can be expanded to six times its original size. As it is stretched, the slits become diamond shaped, a sort of designer scar. It's very ingenious.

February 21

I think I'm watching a parade. So much happens so fast, and there is no time to react or process. I'm living all sorts of adventures, but they hardly seem to be impacting.

March 12

Our team is treating a patient in her thirties with breast cancer. She's had all the therapies available. She's not going to survive this illness. I actually heard one of my peers say to her, "Quit feeing sorry for yourself. We all have to die sometime." Granted, she is not dying very gracefully, but I went back to the room later and apologized for his simplistic, sadistic approach. She told me her sister had died of the same thing four months before.

CHAPTER 11

Lessons about Life

March 21

Life on the ward, be it pediatrics, surgery, internal (infernal) medicine, or whatever, is pretty intense. Today, I actually got to spend a day in the library. There's so much I need to learn to take better care of my patients, and no time to ask anyone. Asking a team member, especially on rounds, runs the risk of being answered with a command to bring back a definitive current answer on the issue by tomorrow.

My present passion is colon cancer. Much of what I read at least mentioned diet as a possible factor in the prevention and causation of colon cancer. Dr. Denis Burkitt is the leading proponent of increased fiber, from grain and potatoes, as a preventative. This advice springs from years of observation, and is not an issue that can be proven by a scientific, prospective randomized, double-blind study. In Africa, bowel cancer is rare, which Burkitt attributes to rapid stool transit time. He's done an extensive study of stools around the world.* If one's stool sinks, one must increase the dietary fiber.

Here's an entertaining piece of information. The chemicals in a bowel movement that give it a foul odor are indole and scatole, the latter being the source of the word "scatologi-

---

*A proper British stool is twice round the bowl and tapered at both ends. An African bushman's stool is heroic.

cal," as in scatological humor, or humor having to do with body products.

Aren't printed words glorious? Why would anyone rob a bank if he could break into a bookstore and read all night?

March 13

I'm on a plastic surgery elective now. One of my original questions about how much of a body does a person need to survive is being answered before my eyes. I wish it weren't. A young woman, too drunk to be hitchhiking, was struck by a passing car. She lost the right leg, and had a broken pelvis. Due to infection and loss of blood supply, we keep carving away, trying to save her life. She is perfectly alert and still willing to live. We took the right pelvis, to get rid of an infection, and part of the left leg, to keep the muscle-break-down products from ruining the kidneys. Now it looks like the left pelvis will have to go. She and her parents are trying to decide if life as a half body will have a quality she can tolerate.

Assisted in the repair of the face of a man in his thirties who wrecked his car to save another driver who was on the wrong side of the road. The accident was at midnight, and he walked about two hours before finding a house. The steering wheel had peeled his nose upward and his cheeks and top lip downward. When the house occupants saw him, they told him to get lost and slammed the door. Their fear or indifference could have cost his life. He finally found help on the highway. He is a very pleasant and positive sort of person. I don't know why he has any respect left for humanity. Claire Boothe Luce said it best, "No good deed goes unpunished."

March 30

I am so tired. Watching medicine behind the scenes, knowing what a poor job is sometimes done, seeing some of the dishonesty, and filling in for irresponsible people is very wearying. I wrote a little poem.

Officially Worn Out

I've been jaded and traded,
My "real self" has faded away.
I'm just walking facts and gruesome acts,
But I just let the music play.

April 30

It's difficult to write during psychiatry because that's what I do all day long. The notes have to be thorough: What they wore, how they sat, what they said, what they thought about what I said, how they said it, why did I think they said it. I saw eight outpatients at a clinic for six weeks. I think they made good progress; only one needs more "work" as we call it. Some nights, I went to the crisis center and learned to answer the suicide line.

Spent a few days on an inpatient ward, a wild and unpredictable place. I like to sit in on what they term "community meeting." It's a combination of group therapy, a courtroom drama and "What's My Line."

At community meeting today, two new patients were looking around the circle of chairs and recognized each other. There was an exuberant reunion; they turned out to be husband and wife. She had left him when quite angry months before, and by the time she came home, he'd been evicted and she couldn't find him.

After we congratulated them, an eighteen-year-old began explaining the great depression he felt over his sister's suicide. The attending psychiatrist kept exploring the subject, and finally another patient elucidated the entire discussion by clarifying that the other guy was not depressed because his sister was dead, but because he hadn't worked up the courage yet to kill himself and she had beat him to it.

Next, the lady sitting next to me explained the origin of intelligent life in the universe, making a pretty consistent reconciliation of *The Bible, The Tibetan Book of the Dead,* and the movie *2001: A Space Odyssey.* Then we had lunch.

For some reason, most people think schizophrenia implies multiple personalities. It actually is a label for persons out of touch with reality. I was interviewing someone whom I was about to diagnose as depressed, because he repeatedly told me everything was fine until the blues came around. The blues had been around for about a year, no one could escape the blues. So I said, in my best reflective tone, "You are really sad a lot."

"Oh, I'm never sad," he replied.

"Then can you explain to me about the blues?"

According to the patient, the Pope's favorite color is blue. The Pope had organized all his friends into a powerful group designed to follow the patient and ruin his reputation. They are the blues. They can control his mind, so he must fight them.

He has no clothes that fit, because, after he buys them, the blues alter them, somehow, to make him look bad. Thank goodness, some friends gave him non-blues pants to wear. This type of schizophrenia is the paranoid type. It is rather common, but fairly treatable with Prolixin. The blues man drives, works, keeps an apartment, and keeps the blues at bay.

I evaluated a woman, age twenty-four, married for a year, whose husband brought her in for treatment of her "seizures." The seizures amounted to tantrums, real foot-stomping, wall-pounding, floor-rolling, screaming-meemee, meat-and-potatoes fits. They occurred when she got angry, after which she would settle down and suck her thumb. The most accurate diagnosis in my manual had to be "inadequate adjustment to adult life."

May 5

Sitting in community meeting on the psych ward, next to a someone who had not spoken since a psychotic break the week before. Someone asked what was going on in the world "outside." I was the only one who had seen the morning paper. I usually didn't contribute, but was asked to share a piece of news. The only story I could remember was about a fellow who had taken a local McDonald's restaurant by storm, and held three people hostage at gunpoint.

"What did he want?" one of the patients asked.

"A hundred thousand dollars," I replied.

The mute psychotic chimed in softly, "And a Big Mac to go."

All the patients and staff laughed, and the discussion headed another direction. I was astonished at the sense of humor that jumped out from under the illness. It was the last thing she said for another week.

For about a week, I have wanted to be a child psychiatrist. Their minds are incredible, their mental illnesses so different from adults'. Most of their problems are social, however. If we could alter the home environment, many of them would improve rapidly.

CHAPTER 12

I Move Up in the Hierarchy

Year Four

July 10

I'm almost in the doctor club. The harassment on rounds now focuses on the third-year students, so I don't spend my study time memorizing "rat facts" to be stored away until called for. This whole year is spent in electives of my choosing, with certain general requirements. The students who already know exactly what they want to do are spending three-quarters of the year doing only that, in various places around the country, to try to impress the powers that be, so they will be chosen for a residency in their chosen field, in their chosen city. I have too many other things I want to learn, so I may not be as competitive when next July arrives.

I selected neurosurgery as my first senior rotation. I haven't learned much brain or spine anatomy, because there is too much work for the sole resident and myself. I have learned an enormous amount about critical care, and dealing with patients and families in very dire circumstances.

Usually, when the brain is injured, a part of the person is lost. In cases of severe damage, when families are waiting for a head-injured person to wake up, I have seen a pattern. First, they say, "Just let him survive. That's all we care about, he has to live." Soon it becomes, "Now, just let him open his eyes."

If the comatose person does become conscious, the next phase of wishing begins with, "Just let him respond, just recognize one of us. We don't care if he's back to normal, just let him see who we are."

When the person begins to follow commands, the bargaining with God, or pleading with whatever power the family believes in, advances to let him talk, let him walk, let him get back to life at home, at work. Unfortunately, the entire sequence rarely happens, the person, for example, plateaus at the "able to watch television" stage, and the family often becomes quite despairing and angry with the team that saved their loved one, only to find him or her in a "persistent vegetative" state.

July 22

Sat with a young man last night who had flipped his truck, and sustained a neck fracture rendering him quadriplegic (paralyzed in all four limbs). When he got the news, he began screaming, "Michael, wake up, wake up!" He was Michael. He screamed all night, demanding that all this be a bad dream. He frequently asked me to kill him, if this was not a bad dream.

I told him my job was to get him through the first part of this horrible experience, and he was free to determine his fate when he'd had time to try to make the emotional adjustment to his loss. I tried to make my answer as compassionate as possible, but it sounded so lame, even to me as I spoke it. He said he wasn't a person any more. I said a person is not his body. A person is not his thoughts. A person is not his feelings. A person is a conscious center of awareness capable of interacting with other conscious centers of awareness; all the rest is just trappings for our use. It didn't sound quite so lame, but I don't know if anything could be said that would be adequate consolation.

August 1

Went on rounds with the chest surgeons today. There was a thirty-eight-year-old man, a friend of a friend of mine, hospitalized with shortness of breath. We put him to sleep this morning to biopsy a lump seen on a chest X ray. It turned out to be a horrible cancer, inoperable and unresponsive to chemotherapy or radiation therapy.

We walked into his room in the evening and the chief of the chest service broke the news in this manner: "You have a bad tumor. There's nothing we can do. We'll let the other tumor doctors see if they can help." Then we all left to finish rounds. I've had enough life experience and sensitivity-oriented role plays in psychiatric rotations that I recognized this as a rather brutal approach to informing the patient of his diagnosis, but thought it must be acceptable since the person in charge was role-modeling it for me. I had seen it before in general surgery. Often, it went more like: "You have a cancer in your ————. We're going to operate tomorrow."

I returned to see how the patient was taking the news, since I knew he was recently divorced and didn't have much support. In addition, he was undergoing one of the largest stresses of his life: being separated from his children.

He was staring at the wall in stunned silence, although an hour had passed since the thoracic tornado had visited his room. I asked if he was okay. He asked me if he had cancer. Recalling the conversation, I realized that only the word tumor had been used. Then he began a litany of technical and prognostic (outcome) questions that I could not answer. About that time, the radiation-therapy physician arrived. She had to suffer the fury of a terminal patient, which would more accurately have been aimed at cigarettes, the cycle of life and death, and a callous surgeon. This gentleman had a short course of radiation and a devastating course of chemotherapy, dying within a month of his admission to the hospital.

It was three years after my involvement in this case before I actually saw adequate and humane cancer counseling in action. The circumstance was a man in his late sixties, who had a biopsy and returned with his wife to get the results. My mentor, Dr. Fred Herzon, asked me to step into his office to learn his method of giving patients terrible news. It was so enlightening to me that I remember it almost verbatim.

Mr. ———, you have a cancer that will most likely cause your death within the next year. (He later said to me, "It's important to use the words cancer and death right away. Most people already know and will respect your honesty.") After you hear that sentence, it's possible you will not remember anything else I say today. It's okay, you are welcome to call back and ask any questions which occur to you.

I want to discuss three options with you. The first is to do absolutely nothing. This should be your decision alone, since we are discussing your life. I'm glad your wife is here, so she can understand that as of this moment, any decision you make about your care is the right decision, because you are the one who should be in control. If you choose to do nothing, let me explain how your death may occur. These cancers cause people to lose their appetites. You can let the natural course of the illness happen and just stop eating. This is not a painful way to die, if it is the death you choose. I want you to know I will keep you comfortable and be there for you, no matter what you choose. It is possible that the cancer will wear into a large blood vessel and you will have a sudden bleed from your neck or mouth. This is very frightening, but not painful. Your family can try to bring you to the hospital, but you may choose to die at home.

The second option is to have some treatments that will possibly increase the length of your life, but probably not the quality of it. (He described some palliative surgical techniques and drug and radiation possibilities).

The third option is a major surgery that will remove your

ability to speak and swallow, and have a less than 5 percent chance of cure. I do not recommend it, since you will probably spend most of the next few months in the hospital, and you will have no social joys when you leave.

Do you have any questions for me?

This amazing, frail-looking couple cried a few tears; then the man said to his wife, "If I start bleeding, you can help me into the bathtub so I won't soil the carpet, and we won't waste a bunch of our savings on hospital care. Think you can do that, Honey?" She thought so. The advising physician warned that when his blood pressure got low enough, he might stop bleeding and would probably be unconscious for up to a day before dying. They spent a few more moments plotting strategies. They said they had made their decisions, thanked us for being so straightforward, and promised to call if anything was needed.

Of course, the entire exchange was only common sense and kindness, but I was still floored. Somehow, I had not been aware that one could give the patients so much control of their destinies. If I say you may choose this death or that death, doesn't it mean I've failed by not stopping death altogether?

I've had many opportunities to extend this compassion to patients. One said I was doctoring "Bernie Siegel style" and gave me his wonderful book *Love, Medicine and Miracles*. From it, I learned more about how medicine should be.

Incidentally, the book that taught me the most facts about medicine is a novel written by Samuel Shem, M.D., entitled *The House of God*. I highly recommend both books.

August 15

I'm getting very interested in delicate surgery, so I tried to do an ear, nose, and throat rotation in Washington, D.C. It was a chance to see how medicine is practiced elsewhere. I arrived there, spent one day on the rotation, and found out my loan was not coming through in time to allow me to survive there, so I saw the sights for three days and came back home. What did I learn in one day? If a cockroach crawls in an ear, it can be drowned in mineral oil, but the swimming motion scratches the ear drum, which is excruciating. Lidocaine, sprayed in the ear canal, numbs the drum and roaches hate it and come flying out backwards. I saw it with my own eyes.

Oh, I also stomped it with my own foot.

I met a woman trying to decide if she wants to live without her larynx (voice box). She has cancer, and has been told, with only radiation treatment, she probably won't survive. She doesn't want to have to speak with a vibrating "electric larynx" or by regurgitating air or by any other ideas the throat surgeons had. It's a major quality-of-life issue for her.

August 22

Rural problems are a little different. My first case on arriving back was to help reattach a woman's thumb bitten off by a horse. About the same time, in the hospital parking lot, a man stepped out of a car, dressed in camouflage with a sleeveless T-shirt and sporting a bandana tied around his brow, in the fashion of Rambo, the fictional tough guy. A fellow getting out of an adjacent vehicle commented, "You don't look like Rambo." I guess the man in costume wasn't as muscularly endowed as Sylvester Stallone. Well, pseudo-Rambo didn't take the assessment very kindly, produced a machete, and gave the critic a few whacks and left. We reattached a few of the critic's fingers and sewed up a head wound. It only took him about forty-five seconds to walk into the emergency room, carrying his own hand parts. What a crazy world.

September 2

I'm doing a "nonclinical" rotation, radiology (X ray reading). I don't see any patients. It's a nice break, but I don't think I could spend my professional life sitting in the dark, hallucinating about shadows on film.

I've agonized over the available choices for residency. There are twenty-three. I've listed the pros and cons over and over, which include lifestyle, length of residency (three to six years), suitability to my personality, competitiveness of the positions, how to do good and well simultaneously. It's maddening. Family practice, emergency medicine, oncology (study of cancer), etc., etc. I can't tell if there is any right answer.

September 15

I have decided to try to get into otolaryngology (ear, nose, and throat surgery) residency, after much soul searching. I'm in the top quarter of my class, which probably isn't good enough, but it feels like a good fit and I will try. This residency requires two years of general surgery first, so if I don't land an ENT spot, I may get to continue in general surgery.

October 25

I did several ENT interviews. The final date of the decision-making process is December 15, when all the applicants find out if they have been accepted or rejected. In the meantime, I am doing burn and trauma rotation. The hours are ghastly. The stories are heart-rending. Our whole team looks terrible and is constantly sleep deprived.

The burned patients are special. They don't have the kind of illnesses I've taken care of before. They are usually normal, healthy people who have had a terrible mishap. Most seem to have a sense of humor intact, which usually isn't possible for chronically ill folks.

I am following a young man burned in an oilfield fire. I had only seen him in wraps, until today. We went to the tub room, which has a large jacuzzi-like tank, in which we soaked him. He has a 60 percent second- (partial) and third- (full-thickness) degree burn. All the burned areas are scraped to get rid of dead skin and bacteria. It is extremely painful, despite morphine. This fellow sang country-western ballads during the entire scrubdown. Tears ran down my face for the ten minutes I helped, just seeing the pain, and courage.

People do rather unintelligent things occasionally, injuring themselves in the process. One of my present patients was burned after trying to check the level of gasoline in his motorcycle tank, using a cigarette lighter.

October 30

I thought I might get some sleep last night, but the "knife and gun club" downtown had a meeting when the bars closed. Someone brought a large hunting knife to the meeting; unfortunately his opponent brought a 9mm handgun, and shot into his abdomen. He arrived in the emergency room without a blood pressure due to a hole in the large artery en route to a leg. About half of his blood volume had poured into the abdomen. The resident cut into the left chest (the patient was unconscious), clamped across the aorta (large vessel leaving the heart), and shot an ampule of epinephrine and one of calcium straight into the heart. The clamp stopped all blood flow to, and blood loss into, the lower body. As the heartbeat got stronger, it was only circulating blood to the brain, lungs, arms, and heart muscle.

We searched the abdomen for injuries, pressure packed

several large bleeders, and moved the aorta clamp down below the arteries that supply the kidneys. The kidneys should not have the oxygen supply cut off for more than thirty minutes. We patched arteries and clamped veins for an hour. We gave fifteen units of blood. We threw in platelets (cells that cause clotting) and plasma (fluid portion of blood with clotting factors) and he still couldn't be made to clot. I knew when my second shoe filled with blood that we were not going to save his life.

There was a phrase that I think was popularized in the Vietnam conflict: "Kill 'em all; let God sort them out." It expresses the frustration of not knowing who are the good guys and who are the bad guys. The trauma team variant is: "Save 'em all; let the city police department sort them out."

December 2

When I take care of the weekend warriors, as we sometimes call them, they are often unshaven, drunk, and unwashed. Sometimes their feet are so dirty, the socks are chemically bound to the skin of the foot (termed "toxic sock syndrome"). They bite and claw and spit at me while I'm trying to help them. Sometimes they get off of their stretchers to try to finish the fight with the guy on the next stretcher. In order to keep up my enthusiasm for helping these people live to party another day, I try to picture them as the pink, soft baby boys they undoubtedly once were, bouncing on someone's knee.

They seem to value no one's life, least of all their own. I keep trying to understand how such a large segment of our society came to think in these patterns. Besides food, shelter and clothes, we need three things in life. We need someone to love, someone to love us and something meaningful to do.

If a person has neither work nor a loving family, it's no wonder they have nothing to lose. That person is extremely dangerous.

CHAPTER 13

I Discover My Path, Sort Of

December 4
I'm still ambivalent about my future. Even went to a family-practice interview. I cannot make up my mind.

December 5
Dr. Stache and I were running a code in the emergency room. That means someone was calling out drugs to be given. I was squeezing a bag, forcing air into the patient's lungs, the doctor pumping the chest to press the heart against the spinal-column bones to circulate blood. We had already defibrillated (electrically shocked) the heart once. We did it a second time and it began to beat. A code puts people in pretty close proximity. We were all in scrub clothes (the equivalent of green pajamas), which rarely fit well. I continued to do the "bagging" while everyone else began to relax.

I must have been exposing some of my chest, leaning over the patient, going through my code calisthenics. Dr. Stache commented, "Why, Dr. Sparks, why aren't you wearing a bra?" Actually, almost none of the trauma residents or students wore any underwear at all, or it would be covered in blood by the end of the day. The resuscitation room became very silent, the nurses and techs waiting for my answer. They all knew I was seriously considering a surgical career and couldn't afford to make an enemy of an attending. We were all pretty hypersensitive about sexual harassment. If I don't know what to say, I just make it funny. An old joke of my sister's popped into my head: "You know, if you didn't have hands, you wouldn't buy gloves."

The retort was a hit. I never knew if the attending was teasing or moralizing or doing what many trauma surgeons seem to do, which is try to keep some levity in their war-zone lives. By the end of the day, I had been congratulated by quite a few people, who had heard through the grapevine that I had been glib with a person in power, and gotten away with it. I have not been able to analyze the meaning of the interaction.

December 13

I found out that I was not accepted in any ENT program for the coming year. It's okay. I am a person who believes things that are meant to be, will happen. I went to Dr. Stache for advice. To my great surprise, he said I'd make a good surgery resident, had worked hard, been able to think while exhausted, and didn't panic in high stress. He said he'd make some inquiries. The next day the surgery department chairman called me to his office and offered me a position.

I am living a charmed life. About a hundred people are clambering for one of the four positions available here. Now, they will only have three positions to fight over. It's an understatement, but I must say my joy is great.

December 24

I am doing an internal-medicine elective. I feel as if I am driving in the slow lane again. The most exciting admission this week was a seventy-five-year-old man who fainted while his daughter was cutting his hair. At least, I think he fainted. It was overly warm in the house, and he had been drinking. I haven't found a seizure disorder or a stroke or myocardial infarction (heart attack). Perhaps my discharge diagnosis shall be "Samson and Delilah syndrome."

January 23

It's time to do another small-town rotation in rural America. My preceptor is a one-hundred-pound genius ball of fire running a National Health Service Corps clinic. I call him "Big Al." He is all this community has in terms of health care provider, so he has taught me an unbelievably wide variety of procedures and therapies. In one day, we did a vasectomy, relocated a dislocated shoulder, and diagnosed three different rashes. The shoulder was great. We basically got the patient stoned on Demerol, so he could relax his muscles, tied a twenty-five-pound weight to his forearm, and let gravity do the rest. When that didn't quite do the trick, Big Al put his little stockinged foot in the fellow's axilla (armpit) and wrestled that shoulder joint into submission. My role was to wrap a sheet around the patient's waist and lean the opposite direction, pulling the sheet. What a circus, and it worked!

January 26

I continue to be unhappy about the care I am able to give my obese patients. I can't find their veins, to draw blood or give fluids, can't feel a uterus, a liver, a spleen, a lymph node, a pulse, or a thyroid. I know that many people have eating disorders because of terrible childhoods. Their addiction is as difficult to treat as any other. I wonder if the lifespan of obese persons is shorter, not only because of an overworked heart, but because we physicians can't make some dangerous diagnoses as early on them.

I examined a very large man who had been in an auto accident. Ideally, I would like to have done a computed axial tomogram (CAT scan) of his neck, because he had a lot of pain in it. The CAT-scan table moves, and it will only move three hundred pounds.

This fellow happened to be an opera singer on his way home from a performance, when he somehow steered his car into a fire hydrant. He was only going about five miles an hour, but his neck got quite a snap. I asked if his car was ruined. He said the front end was fine, but he was afraid he had "totalled" the inside with his bouncing. He had no nerve weakness, so we sent him away in a neck brace. I want the whole world to be okay, I just don't know how to make it so. I want everyone to be so well and so safe that doctors everywhere have to look for work in a different field.

I've finished my rural rotation, having diagnosed scabies (parasite that lives under the skin), lice, AIDS, hepatitis, amebic dysentery, and every common childhood contagious illness. I learned to wash my hands.

February 9

Some visits to the doctor are social. I began interviewing a small elderly woman, who informed me she knew my attending's ex-wife. She confided in me, stating the woman was a "B-I-T-C-you-know-what," and that the office nurse he had before this one was an overbearing know-it-all. Those were her responses to my question, "How long have you had this breathing problem?"

Some visits call for social commentary. I went to the emergency room to evaluate a woman who had been beaten by her husband. He had brought her in, worried that she had a broken jaw. I have taken care of many women assaulted by their loved ones. I usually don't get to meet the perpetrator.

He explained rather casually that she had been mouthing off and he had lost his temper, but now he was in control again. It had happened the night before. She had lost consciousness for about five minutes. Her face was quite bruised and swollen. I felt for broken bones. I checked to see if her teeth fit together. I requested X rays of her jaw and her neck bones. I called the resident to review the case with me, and make sure the films showed no bones broken. We like to monitor, or have the families monitor, for twenty-four hours anyone who has lost consciousness. They may have bleeding or swelling in the brain. That amount of time had nearly passed since the injury, so the patient was free to go.

I went to discharge the woman and asked if I could speak to her alone. The husband said, "No." I could have had him removed by our security men, but the woman said it was fine. "What's bothering me," I said, "is that your husband gave me the entire history of what happened. I really want to hear it from you." She looked at him for permission and received a shrug.

"We argue a lot," she said, "mostly about money. He pushes me around sometimes. Once in a while, he slaps me, but that's like most couples, I guess. Last night it happened pretty much like he said, things just got out of hand."

"Did you fight back?"

"Oh, no!"

"Did you call the police?"

"Well, actually, the fight started at home. I was on my way out for groceries with the kids. He was really angry, told me to leave the kids with him and hurry back so we could finish the discussion. After I got to the store, in a few minutes, he came into the store. I guess he changed his mind. He started the discussion again, and it got more heated, and he flew into a rage, hitting me. My son was really frightened, and he screamed for someone to call the police. Most of the people there know us, so they just went about their business."

The wife was telling this so matter of factly, as if life was supposed to be like this. It is illegal for one person to beat another. Wives are not property. The veneer of civilization seemed so thin on the husband sitting before me, but he displayed no embarrassment or regret concerning this.

"Then what happened?"

"I guess that's when I passed out. He carried me to the car, and the kids watched me until I woke up. They said it was about five minutes. When we got home, he apologized, and asked me not to call the police, because it's only a misdemeanor, and the punishment is a fine, and we don't have enough money as it is."

It occurred to me no one was going to confront this man, who had committed a criminal act and was not going to be held accountable. I decided to do it, although it is frightening. If he got upset, it was clear he had no personal commitment to refusing to act violently in his relationships, and I was about to enter into a relationship with him. If he chose to act violently towards me, he could clearly take out an eye or bite off a finger of mine before I could get any help.

I'm not saying I was being heroic. I just wanted to satisfy my curiosity, maybe do some educating in a psychological arena, which might prevent a future medical problem. I was angry with him for not having learned yet to be angry without using his fists. I was angry with her for not valuing herself enough to disallow this type of abuse.

"How do you feel about all of this?" I asked the husband.

"Well, I'm sorry. I did bring her here. I'll have to pay a doctor bill; that's a punishment."

"Are you concerned that you hurt another human being?" I said, avoiding the words "wife" and "woman," thinking it might have more impact.

"You didn't find anything broken, right? So, I know, from the fights I've been in with my own friends and enemies, that getting punched is tolerable."

"It's true, you didn't break her jaw. I suspect you broke

something harder to heal. Her trust. Her warm feelings about you have got to be pretty bruised," I said. He was glaring at me, becoming red in the face and clenching his fists. "I think you are getting angry with me. You have every right to get angry and to tell me you are angry. You can shout and stomp and express it all you want. You do not have the right to act on your anger by hurting me, however."

"That's just your opinion," he said, getting to his feet.

"I'm not trying to contradict you," I reasoned, "but it is not just my opinion. It is the absolute basis for the freedom we have in America and would be the key to world peace. I need to say one more thing, to both of you. A woman in her home has the right to be safe. All people, in or out of their homes, need to be safe."

I gave her the card containing information about the domestic-violence shelter. I gave them both the cards with the information about the counselling available in their part of town. I tried to maintain some rapport with both of them, since I believe treating people with dignity and respect may inspire that mind-set in them, but it doesn't mean I didn't want to hurt him, and rescue her and the children from such a situation. Any time there is enough anger to hit someone, there is a possibility of death. Inability to express anger in a nonviolent way must not be minimized.

This case has weighed heavily on my heart. I'm trying to understand the new term "feminist." If a "racist" promotes one race over another, and fascists and communists promote their "isms" over others, then does a feminist promote the causes of women over the causes of men? Is there no such thing as a "masculist" because the causes of men have been promoted more than others through history? It's true I work in a male-dominated field, but I'm still struggling for some understanding of these issues.

I don't want a matriarchy. I don't want a patriarchy. I want a "uni-archy" where we promote human issues over all race, gender, age, weight, and whatever other issues exist. I don't know how to create such an utopia, except to keep talking about it.

Have I ever mentioned that complex, difficult questions have simple, easy-to-understand, wrong answers?

CHAPTER 14
Rolling Home

March 1

Had lunch with a lot of bored, burned-out medical personnel. Cafeteria food is hardly fit for human consumption. We are spending much of our time taking care of people trying to self-destruct. The chief resident decided to have some fun over the noon hour. He called the paging operator, and had her call overhead for "Dr. Rubin, Dr. Billy Rubin." Bilirubin is a yellow pigment in the blood. We were so tired that we found it much more clever and funny than it actually was, I'm sure. We paged "Dr. Bumin, Dr. Al Bumin." Albumin is a protein, the equivalent of egg white, in the blood. Then there was "Miss Sarah Bellum, Miss Sarah Bellum, please call neurology." Cerebellum is the back part of the brain. My personal favorite came from Shannon, the urology tech who created "Myra Mains, Myra Mains, please call pathology immediately." (My remains, in case you didn't get it.)

March 3

I get to do something out of the ordinary. I asked permission from the graduation committee if I could write a curriculum for myself for this month. I want to learn about acupuncture. In our institution there is a physician who also is a licensed acupuncturist. We don't know how a lot of medicine works, so I don't want to exclude any possibilities that might be helpful. I watched an operation performed using hypnotism and acupuncture for anesthesia. I was impressed. Acupuncture has been practiced in Asia for thousands of years. It is not "mind over matter" because it is equally successful when used on children and animals.

My project consists of selecting patient volunteers with pain problems. I couldn't get enough interested arthritis sufferers, so I chose menstrual-cramp subjects. Similar studies have been done in Yugoslavia and China. They claim success, but my study has a special twist: I'll be drawing blood to look for endorphins—the body's morphine—to see if I can show that chemical as the source of the pain relief. My control group is women who will be receiving sham or fake acupuncture. The needles will be placed off the prescribed meridians, and will not go as deep.

April 10

I'm confused. All my fake acupuncture patients got better and none of my real ones did. No one knew which she was receiving. Now I've got all these vials of blood, waiting to be tested for endorphins, but I doubt if anybody will be much interested in my article, which would imply that I have come up with a pain relief system better than the ancient technique. I'll follow the results for a few months, maybe they'll reverse themselves.

I learned an enormous amount of alternative medicine. It doesn't lend itself to scientific analysis very well, so I am quite disappointed that my endorphin question will not likely be answered this time around. I learned to identify 9 of the 365 points and can stick them with a vigor. There are twelve major lines and eight extra lines of energy, called meridians. When these energies get blocked, release is accomplished with a needle, or pressure, or heat, or electricity.

Are these energies electrical, hormonal, mystic? We know not. Complex, difficult questions have . . .

April 15

The end is in sight. There's a light at the end of the tunnel; I just hope it's not a train. In a month I will have gainful employment, and a long-term goal met, but in the meantime, I have one last rotation, emergency medicine.

It feels like a car wash; we spiff them up and send them home or into the bowels of the hospital, and don't know what happens afterwards. Heck, if I know whether or not it turned out to be gonorrheal pelvic inflammatory disease. It didn't seem like an ovarian torsion or ectopic (tubal) pregnancy. The gynecology team will know by this time tomorrow.

I see three or four people an hour. Some serious, some who aren't sick, some who are very funny. I treated a man today whose entire scalp, eyelids, and upper lip swelled to about three times normal. It was a reaction to the hair dye he had used. After we loaded him up with epinephrine, steroids, and diphenhydramine, his lip size decreased enough for him to ask me if the gray hair was gone.

I checked his old records. The same thing had happened several years before. I guess beauty knows no pain.

May 14

In ten hours I will no longer be a medical student. I'm so delirious that I can hardly think. It's been the greatest honor, and a total nightmare. Some of the gains and loses have been disclosed in my journal. I'm sure the tempering of naïveté and idealism occur as rites of passage in most adult lives, but they have seemed quite dramatic for me in the last four years.

May 15

I'm "here." I'm a doctor. Will I think clearly? Will I kill people? One certainty in medicine: one can never know enough to be adequate. I'm already wishing I could be alive in two hundred years to see what the alternatives will be to what we do. We find a cancer and chop it out, poison it with chemotherapy, burn it with radiation. It's all so crude, but it's all we've got. I want to be a magician, not a physician. I want the faith healers to walk through my intensive care units touching people, and walk out the doors with the patients walking beside them, telling me to get lost, that there is no need for me there.

Perhaps that time will come. It will mean there is no work for policemen, no need for soldiers as well. It will likely mean that we have stopped eating processed pseudo-food, irradiated, waxed, insecticide-covered, nutrition-depleted produce, steroid- and antibiotic-injected meat, which was an unnecessary part of our diets anyway.

Until all that happens, I'll just keep on trying to save lives and alleviate suffering, and hoping that sometimes these two things go hand in hand.

Epilogue

Update 1996: I worked as a traveling doctor, filling in for missing physicians for several years, doing a great deal of recreational travel in between. I spent a lot of time learning about the world and our potential for peace. I have a private practice and a full, happy life. I'm not impaired. I don't think I'm greedy. There are still plenty of sick folks.

References

Barrows, H. and R. Tamblyn. *Problem-Based Learning: An Approach to Medical Education.* Med. Educ. Ser.: Vol. 1. New York: Springer Pub., 1980.

Sagan, C. *The Dragons of Eden.* New York: Random House, 1977.

Seigel, B. *Love, Medicine and Miracles.* New York: Harper & Row, 1986.

Shem, S. *The House of God.* New York: Dell, 1981.

Stone, W.G. *The Hate Factory.* New York: Dell, 1982.